KETTLEBELL

Kettlebell Workouts for Building Massive Muscles
and Gaining Strength

(Healthy and Fitness of Kettlebell Training)

Corey Farmer

I0135118

Published By Corey Farmer

Corey Farmer

Kettlebell: Kettlebell Workouts for Building Massive Muscles and Gaining Strength (Healthy and Fitness of Kettlebell Training)

ISBN 978-1-77485-385-6

Legal & Disclaimer

TABLE OF CONTENTS

Introduction

Kettlebell is among the exercises that people consider interesting and cool. If you've not experienced the kettlebell before then you're probably wondering about what it looks like. It's actually quite simple. It's a cannonball in black with a handle made from iron. Although there are many other exercise tools can be used to meet your goals for health Kettlebells offer advantages for health should you decide to integrate it into your exercise routine.

The reason kettlebells are exercises so mystical is in their roots. They gained popularity in Russia during the early 18th century. At the time the kettlebell was employed as a counterweight when measuring items like cereals or other dry goods.

The farmers began battling each other to carry the largest kettlebells and, in the end, they managed to find their route to powerful circus masters. Following after the Second World War, the Soviet Red Army took up kettlebells to train their soldiers.

In the 1970s, and later after the 1970s, kettlebell lifting was declared as an official sport in the 1970s.

Although kettlebells have been in use across the US for more than 100 years, they've seen their own share of revival and finally made their way into gyms or fitness store. They consist of a bell the handle, and the horns. The bell, in this instance is the cannonball shape round weight. The handle is the part that connects the kettlebell, by sliding downwards at each end and is referred to as the Horns.

This is the design that makes the kettlebell an distinct device. You might be wondering "what is the main difference in kettlebells as opposed to dumbbells?" Well, one important thing to keep in mind is that, in contrast to dumbbells where the handle is connected to two weights equally distributed and sits in the center

The kettlebell's center of gravity is typically off from the handle. This is because it sits a couple of inches from the middle.

It is important to remember that when you use kettlebells, it's extremely easy to grasp it with the handle bell end, bell or the horns. This is the most common way to grasp the kettlebell using its handle. But in specific exercises, like squats for example it is more convenient to hold them with the bells. To get a better grasp on certain poses, like rowing, it is best to keep the kettlebell in the bell the bell. This can be done

as it helps by forcing your hand into a position that makes it squeeze more in order to stop the hand from sliding.

Chapter 1: Shoulders and Arms

If you are just beginning kettlebell training, you should start with kettlebell exercises that work specifically with the arms and shoulders. The exercises below although they can be beneficial for various muscle groups, impact mostly the shoulders and arms. The majority of them are easy to master and learn but some may require some knowledge before they are mastered however, they are all guaranteed to yield benefits that traditional training methods are likely to replicate.

1. The Kettlebell Slingshot

Muscle group to target: Shoulders and Arms

Guide: This fluid exercise is very simple to perform on paper, however it's more difficult to learn as well as master than appears and could require hours of repetition to master. The immediate advantages of this exercise might not be apparent but as you progress you'll notice that your flexibility in your shoulders has improved and strength in your arms has grown.

Start by standing straight and with your shoulders apart. Keep the kettlebell in front of you at approximately an inch above your chest, and then move it behind you. Utilizing the other hand extend your arm behind your back and grasp the weight, making it complete circle back towards your chest. This is a repetition. When you've completed one set, turn how you swing, and continue the exercise. This is a great exercise for your entire upper body, as the movement involved in moving the kettlebell around will work more than just your muscle groups of the arm and shoulder. This exercise can help for your core and your Obliques as well as your back and chest benefitting from the movement.

2. The Kettlebell Military Press

Muscle group to target: Shoulders, arms, and back

Walkthrough The walkthrough is one of the drills which can be accomplished quickly using conventional dumbbells, but it is much more efficient when you use kettlebells. The way that weight is distributed on kettlebells ensures that you pay attention to the way that the weight is acting when performing the press. This ensures that you will get the most out of your workout since you must pay more attention to make sure the weight is working for your benefit.

This is a lot like the traditional dumbbell for the military, it is best to start with, you need to grab the kettlebell and then clean it to an appropriate rack posture (the cleaning exercise will be discussed further throughout this manual). The rack is the position in which the kettlebell is in your hands, bent at the elbow, and your fist placed close to your chest. the weight rests on your forearm and close the body. When you are in the rack posture, you can press the weight up straight while leaning slightly forward. The goal is to ensure the kettlebell's weight is on your back. The

6

weight should be brought down and back to the rack for one repetition. Switch arms at the conclusion of the set, and continue the exercise. If you'd like to add an additional exercise, this set can be completed using two kettlebells at same at the same time.

3. Kettlebell Pirate Ships

Muscle group to target: Shoulders Arms, Back, and Shoulders

Guide: One the well-named exercises this exercise is distinctive due to the fact that after performing several repetitions you'll be able to understand the reason they are named pirate ships. The particular workout is perfect for building strength of your shoulders, and also your back, arms, and obliques, as it works the entire upper body during exercise.

Start by placing your feet just an inch wider than your the shoulder width to. You should hold the kettlebell in both hands and then let the weight hang at the waist, keeping your arms extended. Start by moving the kettlebell in one direction, until it is at approximately head height, while you twist your entire body the exact same way. Keep your eyes fixed on the weight at all times.

The weight should be held at a head high for a few seconds before letting it drop. When it falls, turn your body around in the opposite direction and allow the weight to move with your body in the shape of a pendulum. Once more, lift it to the level of your head, and then keep it there for a few seconds before letting the weight fall back to its starting position. This is a repetition. This workout should be performed with the standard 3 to 5 sets of work out, but it can be performed as a time trial to test not just how long you can last however, but also the number of reps you are able to perform before you become exhausted.

4. Kettlebell High Pull

The target muscle group is Shoulders and Arms

Walkthrough The walkthrough is a fluid-style exercise that is extremely beneficial to master and learn however it might not be as simple as it appears. If explained and demonstrated the high pull appears to be a simple routine to master, however the correct body and form positions can be difficult to master correctly. Proper supervision for the first couple of instances of this routine is advised, particularly for those who are new to the sport, simply to ensure that proper form is properly maintained throughout the entire workout.

For the first step, set your feet shoulder-width apart, and then point your toes toward the outside at a 45-degree angle. Put the kettlebell between your legs and then lower yourself towards it while keeping your back straight throughout the procedure. Take the kettlebell in one hand and then rise to its beginning position, lifting the kettlebell by extending your arm until it is at the shoulder height. Lower the weight back to shoulder level and repeat the exercise with the other hand until you have completed one rep.

The one-arm high pull is described as a transitional move as similar to the kettlebell clean, since it's part of the move utilized to create an accretion of the kettlebell.

5. The Kettlebell Figure 8

The target muscle group is Shoulders, Arms

Walkthrough It is a great illustration of a crossfit-inspired Kettlebell exercise. The figure 8 move was a favorite among the world of street basketball before it became apparent the value of this routine helped to develop muscles in the shoulders and arms. Additionally it was discovered that one positive side effect of this exercise was the strengthening in the muscles of lower back, but it isn't as obvious as the improvement observed in the arms and shoulders of those who practice this type of exercise.

To complete the figure 8 using kettlebells, begin by placing both feet slightly more than hip width apart . Then lower your body to the standing squat. Ensure that your back remains straight. Take the kettlebell in your left hand, then move it along the outside of your left leg, then pass it back through the legs and then to you right-hand. Repeat the process with your right hand in order to finish one repetition. Although you are able to perform 10 to 15 repetitions in the recommended amount, with this workout, occasionally you can do the time trial to determine the length you can take. This is a great exercise for people looking to build strength, particularly in their lower back and arms.

There are plenty of other exercises that concentrate on the shoulders and arms but these are the most effective. After a few weeks of training, these exercises will surely become part of your routine exercise routine. And as time passes, you'll be able to do them for a shorter duration than usual exercises, the advantages of these workouts will show through.

Chapter 2: Kettle Bell Training

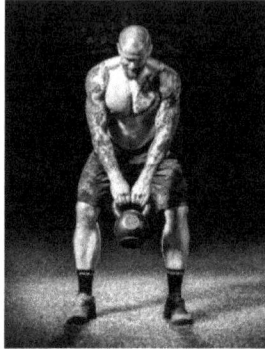

What exactly are Kettlebells?

Kettlebell originated from Russia and was brought to the United States by Russian fitness instructor Pavel Tsatsouline in 2001. Since then, there has been an exponential increase in popularity of kettlebells. There is a good chance that there are over 100,000 people who use kettlebells and this figure will grow in the coming years. The design of the kettlebell reveals its distinctiveness. It's similar to a cannonball that has a a attached handle on the top. In simple terms kettlebells are steel or cast iron free weights where the weight isn't distributed evenly. This allows a person to stay balanced and maintain a steady body during the exercise. Additionally, there are variations of kettlebells that mostly consist of bags filled with water, sand and steel shots.

The main purpose of kettlebell workouts is to strengthen and strengthen grip strength particularly in the shoulders, lower back and legs. The weight of kettlebells can range from 2 pounds to the weight of 106 tons or greater. For exercise, it's essential to choose the correct size kettlebell particularly in the beginning otherwise, it could result in injuries while exercising. Following exhaustive study, it's been found that as a beginner, women should use kettlebells that weigh 8 kg (18 Lb) while males should select sixteen KG (35 kg). However, those who have previous experience with weight training should use a 20 kg (44-pounder) kettlebells for women and 12kg (26-pounder) for males. Furthermore the body shape and the age of an individual are key factors in determining the kettlebell's size, for instance, those who are overweight and have a sedentary lifestyle should use a kettlebells that weigh 26 pounds. (12 kg) for males, and 15 lbs. (6 kg) by females.

Why train with Kettlebells?

In recent years the widespread acceptance of kettlebell training has inspired both genders males and females to utilize kettlebells. However, it's important that the right kettlebell weight is utilized for training or else it could cause an internal or external injuries. Additionally, the main reason to utilize kettlebells for training is because it has the handle more securely than barbells or dumbbells do, helping to develop a solid grip and strong forearms. The reason for this is its distinctive design, which permits an energetic and rapid exercise with a variety of actions.

It lets several muscles work at the same time, that are similar to the real-life exercises that are found in other physical pursuits such as athletics, sports or other. Furthermore, when the primary muscle is that is being worked by a specific movement the weight off-center of the kettlebell can force to increase the force and cause the stabilizer muscle to adjust. This gives every part of your body with an extensive exercise. It is recommended to use dumbbells and kettlebells, you can put together balanced workouts for the whole body. The distinction between dumbbells and kettlebells is that they focus the movements on the primary muscles since the weight is evenly distributed over the area of contact.

Furthermore training with kettlebells is thought to be a more feasible and feasible option for all. This is because they do not require a large amount of area opposed to other fitness equipments such as pull-down lats cable biceps bar as well as hanging leg raise. It is convenient for people and they are able to easily store it in their home or gym, or even take it on trips. It is therefore useful for everyone, from the professional athlete to the person who is sedentary. It is important to select the correct method in accordance with the purpose of the individual.

Benefits of Kettlebell

In recent times many coaches, athletes or personal trainers have turned to kettlebells in their workouts that improves build muscle tone, improve the body's composition, and strength that the muscles produce. Additionally professional athletes and fitness enthusiasts are beginning to realize the value of kettlebell exercise. It helps create stronger joints and is less susceptible to injury through strengthening ligaments and tendons in the human body. In addition the advantages of training with kettlebells are:

Performance improvement: Training using kettlebell trains helps athletes to stand up to the constantly shifting center of gravity. It has been determined that the center of gravity of the kettlebell puts 6-8 inches beyond the grip. it is a mirror of the forces individuals experience in various physical tasks. Thus, kettlebells are able aid in improving general performance for those particularly those who participate in sports.

Exercises for Cardiorespiratory Fitness. The kettlebell exercise can force the muscles of an individual to prepare for breathing, which plays a vital part in the cardio-respiratory fitness. Individuals exercise their arms while in an overhead position, which permits the muscles involved in breathing to participate in the muscular movement.

Learning Time our current world, everyone is working the same amount of time. Therefore it is essential to do exercises that take less time however are more efficient. Training with kettlebells can help people cut down on time spent using their focus to other goals like strategies, skills rest, and recovery. This results in the ability to work out quickly and efficiently because it blends the benefits of fitness training, anaerobic as well as aerobic exercise, and flexibility.

Energy Output main reason to use kettlebells to exercise is the fact that it allows you to make movements over a longer duration of time. This leads in power endurance. Power endurance refers to the capacity to sustain rapid muscle contractions for an extended time. It's also a great technique for those who are aware of their weight and wish to shed fat. Apart from that it aids athletes and decides who wins the sport.

Uniqueness: As mentioned earlier the distinctive shape of kettlebells allows for traditional skills such as kettlebell juggling, which is different from traditional weightlifting exercises. Furthermore, it assists to achieve a greater range of motion, which improves the flexibility of the workout.

Hinge Pattern A hinge pattern is regarded as a pattern that is efficient for those seeking strength and fitness, such as athletes. Kettlebell allows people to swing, which increases the overall athleticism. Furthermore, the swing is an exercise tool that aids many different fields, such as basketball players that want to increase their vertical leap or to teach an athlete to utilize the hips. Thus, by using kettlebells, individuals are able to learn how to create the perfect pattern

Cost-effectiveness: Kettlebell are durable as they are made from steel or cast iron which allow users to use them for long periods of time without needing to be replaced. Furthermore, because of their the widespread popularity, it's easily available at any of the retailers and does not cost a lot such as one kettlebell will cost less than $100. Therefore, individuals based on the type of their physique and needs can buy a variety of sizes of kettlebells at reasonable cost. Additionally it's portable, and users can take it to various locations.

Training with kettlebells is an athletic activity that helps individuals to develop abilities and strength within the body. Furthermore, it permits the development of various athletic traits like strength as well as flexibility, balance endurance, coordination, and of course stamina for the person.

Strong forearms and a strong grip The handle of kettlebells is made from a sturdy material, making it a strong equipment when compared with dumbbells. This allows you to build a sturdy grip as well as powerful forearms. Since the core of the kettlebell is gravity, that is typically moved by exercise of grip. This causes a mixture of static and dynamic muscle contractions that manage the movement of the mass center.

A decrease in body fat: Today women, particularly females, are conscious of their weight and desire to reduce body fat as well as inches around their waists and thighs. They also want to slim their arms. Thus, for overweight people , kettlebell exercise is an effective method of burning excess fat. Since kettlebells increase the metabolic rate of an individual through a vigorous training. The result is a decrease in weight loss. To achieve the desired level it is essential to create a routine to working out daily and include the highest repetition of compound movements. The most common kettlebell exercises are the reverse lunge and shoulder press.

Training for Strength: Kettlebell aims to build strength, not just focusing on muscles. This is accomplished by the growth in muscle mass by performing full-body functional moves. This means that women who don't want to build muscle but want to build their muscles are able to use kettlebells in their training.

Safety Precautions

As mentioned earlier kettlebell training comes with many advantages because of its distinctive qualities. But, there are some guidelines that one has to follow, especially when he is just beginning in kettlebell instruction. This is because it's a demanding exercise that requires complete focus. If someone performs kettlebell exercises in a wrong or unsafe manner , then it could result in injuries or thoughts of delusions. Additionally, being distracted and exhausted by the kettlebell exercise is not going to produce the desired results. It is therefore essential to master the movements and practice them properly to avoid injury. Here are a few safety guidelines which will ensure an enjoyable workout with kettlebells.

Size of Kettlebell The first aspect of weight-training is to choose the appropriate size kettlebell. This means that how heavy the kettlebell has to be suitable. According to the general rule most men will select heavy kettlebells, while women prefer lighter kettlebells. When you say right size, it means that the user can hold the handle correctly so that it is able to be held with both hands , without it overhang. To achieve this the handle must have a large enough to be able to hold it with both hands. If the grip size isn't sufficient, there is a chance that when you swing it, the kettlebell can fall or moves in a different direction, which could hurt anyone. In order to prevent this from happening, individuals particularly novices should choose a kettlebells made of the same part of the material.

Body posture The most important thing is to make sure that posture and posture of your body is in a proper position during kettlebell exercises. First of all, the force generated by the kettlebell must be concentrated in the hips and not by the side of the body. A neutral spine is the best way to ensure posture, and that is why it is important to ensure to ensure that there is an even line from the shoulders to head. One of the ways to keep straight backs are to stand on your feet, with the shoulders should be wide apart , and arms pointing to the sides. Additionally, the focal point of the eyes is an area of approximately six feet in front of the individual sitting standing on the floor, keeping the head and neck in a neutral position. In addition in order to extend to the back of your legs, allow the arms to follow the hips like a person moves backwards from the chair.

Swing: To prevent any injury to the body, nobody who begins kettlebell exercise should take the kettlebell and begin swinging. To get it set up, start with the kettlebell approximately one foot ahead then grab it and then throw it back. It should be like the way a person would walk in a football.

Shoes: In general the majority of people don't look at their clothes during exercise, especially footwear. However, it's been found that wearing inappropriate footwear, such as running shoes, could cause knee injuries as it could push the knee. Therefore, the best kind of footwear for kettlebell exercise is flat-soled footwear to ensure your stability as well as grip to the ground.

Wrist Positioning During a kettlebell exercises, proper wrist positioning is essential to avoid any injury. In order to prevent injury, wrists must be straight, without bending them to prevent additional strains during exercise.

Breathing: The aim of these exercises is not to cause a person to become anxious, hence it is suggested to hold the breathing to ensure safety for kettlebells. In order to do this, the pressure that you put on your spine needs to be controlled. This will also help keep your spine safe by breathing in order to tighten the abdominal muscles. It will take some time and effort to master this technique since it is distinct from regular breathing.

Plenty of space: Alongside these methods, it is essential to conduct kettlebell exercises in a safe space since swinging movements require plenty of space where there are no obstructions to. Outside, exercise is highly recommended but it is vital to make sure that the floor isn't slippery or uneven, in order to avoid any injury.

Kettlebell Swing

The kettlebell can be utilized for different purposes based on the requirements. It's not only about swinging the kettlebell up and down. It involves many kettlebell swings, and should be executed correctly to reach the goal you want to achieve. Here are the easy steps to follow when swinging a kettlebell

First step: the first step is standing with your feet wide apart and hold kettlebells that have one foot ahead of the ground. Then, bend at the waist and grasp the handle of the kettlebell using both hands. The palms should face the body while the body should sit in line with the ground.

Second Step: The 2nd step is to pull your shoulders backward and downward in the in a downward and backward. Support the core prior to commencing the swing. Keep these posture cues throughout the entire set.

Step 3: After the posture is established raise the kettlebell with a the correct grip and swing it between your legs. When swinging it is essential to keep the back straight and the neck straight. Additionally, knees must be slightly bent when swinging.

Step 4 Step 4: During the swing the hips must be pushed with force to move the kettlebell upwards. It is essential that the kettlebell remains in control , and not be higher than shoulders. To achieve this, the kettlebell should be controlled with arm.

Step 5: Now let the kettlebell to swing up and back up between the legs. Control it's descent, keeping your core engaged. Continue to the next rep immediately after the kettlebell is lower.

Step 6: In the last repetition, let the kettlebell move back and forth through the legs. After that, put it to the left of the ground.

Chapter 3: Utilizing the Russian Kettlebell To Get in Shape

Kettlebells, that came from Russia is among the most efficient fitness tools you can have at workplace or at home. Many fitness experts say that you can reach all your fitness goals with this basic and affordable exercise tool. The book does more than just say that we can do it, but we'll show you how to achieve it.

Before we get to the specific exercises you can perform Let's first talk about why you should pick the kettlebell over other exercise equipment are featured in commercials on TV.

It's not expensive

One of the main reasons to buy a kettlebell is the low cost. The kettlebell you are using today is going to last for all of the time. In contrast to the machines for workouts that are found in gyms, your kettlebell isn't likely to break or malfunction. Kettlebells of good quality also won't get rusty. This means they'll remain in good shape even after sweat has been dripping over them for the past decade.

It's easy to use and to store

In contrast to barbells and dumbbells, you don't have to adjust the weights of your kettlebell each time you alter your workout routine. Every kettlebell is equipped with a particular weight. This means that you are able to quickly grab them in your exercise schedule and begin working out. Because you do not need to worry about iron plates, you'll be more comfortable putting them away after workouts.

It is used to exercise your entire body

Many people believe kettlebells are just like dumbbells. If you read more about this guide, however you'll discover that the exercises kettlebells allow you to perform are more varied than dumbbells. It is possible to make use of kettlebells for more than fitness but also for increasing your cardiovascular fitness. Exercises that make use of kettlebells additionally utilize larger muscle groups than the routine workouts performed using barbells. This is mainly used for isolating muscles. With kettlebells, you can make the option of separating the muscle group you want to isolate or perform a variety of muscles at the same time.

Its ergonomic design is reminiscent of carrying objects from your daily life

We typically carry the kettle ball the same manner as we carry groceries in plastic bags or the briefcase. The position of the wrist and suspended arms that are used to carry the kettle allows us to train on the same muscle movements we perform every day when perform our daily tasks. The use of kettlebells will help us become more effective in everyday tasks. This is the reason women and men alike need to start using kettlebells in their routine workouts.

Chapter 4: Intermediate Exercises

Intermediate exercises are best performed by people who have had many kettlebell classes for beginners. Intermediate exercises are physically demanding and require more expertise.

Kettlebell figure 8 goals

The main focus is Back, abdominals, arms

Keep your legs slightly larger than the hip distance. Reduce yourself to a squat posture and ensure that you maintain your spine straight with your shoulders elevated. Take one kettlebell in your left hand, and then swing it toward your left leg , then back between your legs. The kettlebell is passed to your right hand and then swing it to the right side of your leg. The movement is like a classic basketball exercise. Do as many repetitions as possible in the time allotted.

Advanced windmill for kettlebells

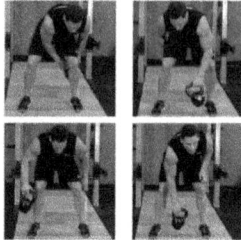

The main focus is the hamstrings, abdominals, glutes, shoulders

Place one kettlebell on your head using only one arm. Make sure the kettlebell is locked and then push your butt in to the opposite direction as the kettlebell is moving. Make sure you keep your working arm behind you. Move your feet 45 degrees to the side of the arm which is holding the kettlebell. lower your body until you stop at the lower end. Then reverse the movement back to the position you started from.

Kettlebells One Leg Dead Lift

The main targets are glutes, hamstrings and lower back.

Use one hand. The leg you lift isn't situated on the opposite side as the hand in the position of holding it. Maintain your knees bent, and do a single leg dead lift by bent your hips while extensing your other leg behind to ensure stability and support. Reduce the kettlebell to the point that it's close to the ground. Then, stop for a second and then return to the beginning position.

One-arm kettlebell jerk

The main targets are calves, shoulders and the triceps

Take one kettlebell and hold it by the handle. The kettlebell should be pulled towards your shoulder by stretching your arms across your hips and legs. Place the kettlebell in the shoulder's back. Your wrist should be rotated with your palms facing towards the forward.

Lower your body, bend your knees, maintaining your torso upright. Reverse the motion quickly and leap to generate momentum. While you jump, you can push the kettlebell up by extensing your arms. Utilize your body to move your weight. Squat back to a standing position, keeping the kettlebell above you. Then return to the standing position. Lower your weight prior to doing another set.

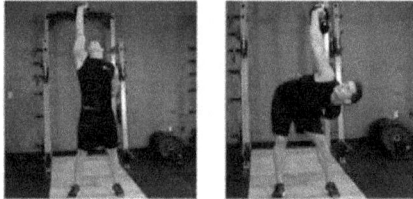

Leg over floor press

Goals: chest, shoulders and the triceps

Lay on the floor you hold a kettlebell in your chest. Spread one leg across your other. Bring your free arm out to the side to provide assistance. You can hold the kettlebell with your elbow resting in a flat position on the ground. Lengthen your arm above your head and then hold it for a few seconds. Reduce your arm until the point reaches the ground. Make sure you keep the kettlebell on your elbow. Repeat this several times.

Alternating kettlebell row

The focus is on the middle back and biceps

Two kettlebells should be placed on your feet. Lean slightly, and push your butt forward to the maximum extent you can. Make a bending motion to grab both kettlebells using the handles. The kettlebell is lifted while you hold one to the other. Reduce your shoulder blade as you extend your elbows. Pull the kettlebell towards your core. The kettlebell will slowly lower and repeat the motion using the other arm.

Kettlebell sumo high-pull

Goals: back, arm and shoulders

Place your feet in a straight line. Put an kettlebell on your foot. Take the kettlebell in both hands. Maintain your knees bent, and you are able to move your legs back. Bring the kettlebell up towards your shoulders as you raise your knees. Gradually raise your elbows. Keep in mind that the force should be taken out of the hips. Maintain your core active all the duration. The kettlebell should be lowered and then repeat the exercise.

Two Kettlebell Front Squat

The goal is to get Legs back

Take two kettlebells and place them on your shoulders. Squat, pressing your heels against the ground, and then pulling your hips forward. Be sure your hips are in line with the ground. Return to the beginning position, and then do 15 repetitions.

Chapter 5: What to Select Your Kettlebells

With the knowledge we have gained about many things about the kettlebell's history and development over time If you're considering buying one, you're now an integral part of the history. One of the biggest difficulties with buying exercise equipment is the idea that one size fits all. Most people simply stroll through the aisle or the showroom at their local sports goods store and choose their first item they come across. They've not done any study on the type of exercise equipment they'll need according to their body type as well as their strengths, limitations and other interests. All of these aspects need to be considered for equipment to be utilized for the long run.

It's worse that buyers will purchase items online, but not have any means of knowing whether it's appropriate for them. When something arrives that isn't an appropriate size, it is removed. I don't want you make the same mistake with your kettlebell. I encourage you to be patient learn about the kettlebell, before you select the one that's most suitable for your needs. I do not recommend the impulse purchase here. There's plenty of variation within these items of equipment and you can see this when you test various kinds.

Consider it as the bowling ball. If you bowl it is not common to take any random ball and begin throwing it across the lanes. If you do, then you've probably not had much success. If you want to be successful at playing it is essential to choose the ball that has right dimensions of openings that fingers will be able to effortlessly slide in or out. Additionally, you must select the weight that is comfortable for you. For certain people the color can be a factor. How can you tell what kettlebell is best for you? Let's discover.

ANATOMY OF A KELL

The fundamental structure of kettlebells is quite simple. They have a cylindrical shape with an extra handle. In addition the kettlebell is different in the numerous shapes and sizes it is available in. Most kettlebells are made of stainless steel or cast-iron since these tend to last longer and are less likely to break down. There are kettlebells coated with vinyl for those who prefer. Some come with distinctive designs such as those with a gorilla-themed face. Additionally, kettlebells that have an adjustable handle can be a good option too.

This may not sound to be a huge deal at first but they can have a major impact in the course of various exercises. It is crucial to feel at ease using your kettlebell for the best results and to feel secure. The last thing I would like is to see you purchase one that isn't comfortable and then you hurt your self.

There are some simple exercises that are able to be done using any kettlebell. These are very easy moves that require only a minimal interaction with the actual kettlebell. Single-leg deadlifts with single-arms and the slingshot is only a few exercises which can be performed regardless of what kind of kettlebell you've got. If you plan to stay with these basic exercises, then this might not be as important. However, the decision you make is vital especially if you intend to go for some intense exercises, which you will eventually. In a nutshell the kettlebell's classic design looks like a miniature cannonball that has an handle.

THE BEST KELLELL for YOU

When picking a kettlebell it's important to select one that isn't damaging the wrists of your forearms shoulders or elbows. The kettlebell will be used on your muscles throughout all workouts, therefore great precautions must be taken. Also, weights that have incorrect handles can break the hands of your hands severely. The two top kinds of kettlebells available on the market are competition kettlebells and cast-iron kettlebells. Both of them will provide immense benefits when you be serious about your training.

The competition kettlebells are uniform in size for all sizes. That means the kettlebell will be the same size between the handle and the cylinder regardless of the weight, whether 8 or 16 kilograms. In many instances there are competitions that are differentiated by colors that are based on international norms. The specific hue of the object will indicate the weight. The kettlebells of this kind are durable because they are made of steel. They're a good choice for those who plan to take competitiveness seriously.

The benefit that the kettlebell for competition gives you is the consistent training and competing. When training using a kettlebell for competition, you can feel the sensation it creates on your wrists. It's the same sensation you experience when you use any kettlebell that is used in competition. Whatever the weight of the equipment is it will be simple to adjust to since the size won't alter. In any professional sports, athletes must be as close as they can to the setting they'll be competing in, as well as the equipment they'll use. For instance, track athletes are likely to try running the track they'll use in competition in the most efficient way possible. This is similar to the kind of advantage you gain with kettlebells used in competition. Similar to having an advantage on the field at home.

These kettlebells come with handles that are small, with a limited space between them. This keeps your hands from sliding side-to-side and causing blisters and burns to the skin. The downside is the fact that just one hand can be able to fit onto the handle. Except if you happen to have hands that are small. I'm talking about extremely, small hands. A lot of kettlebell-related exercises that are important require two hands. With an Olympic kettlebell they aren't feasible. Your workout routine is severely restricted due to the numerous beneficial exercises that aren't in the exercise.

But it's fine because you will still be able to enjoy a fantastic exercise. If you're looking for more variety, we offer an alternative that is great. The cast iron kettlebells can be made by using one piece of steel that is consistent throughout. The physical size of the kettlebell varies based on weight, not unlike the type used in competition. This can make it challenging to keep a consistent training routine and competition. If your primary goal isn't competing, it might not be an issue for you.

The kettlebell in cast iron comes with handles that are larger, which will make it easier to choose from a variety of exercise routines you have at your disposal. It's now possible to utilize two hands which is a great benefit to begin with, since some new workout routines require two hands to complete. The cast iron kettlebell might be the better choice for those who are new to the world due to the variety of uses it offers. Additionally, learning the fundamentals of this part of the kettlebell generally requires two hands. So should you opt for an competition kettlebell right from the beginning your foundation won't be strong. This could result in problems for you later. It's not just that you won't perform to your maximum ability, you also be at risk of major injuries. If you're a beginner stay with cast iron for the moment.

For the experienced user with experience, the competition kettlebell is an excellent choice. Switch from the cast iron kettlebell to the competition once you are comfortable and will be able to add numerous exercises. When you do change gears the two options are employed to get the most varied workouts as you can. If you're determined to take your kettlebell workout to the highest stage The competition kettlebell is the best way to take your training to the next level.

The next important consideration you should make consider the amount of weight that is suitable for you. Similar to any other exercise it's essential to begin slowly and gradually increase the intensity to avoid unnecessary pain and injuries. The weights that kettlebells are typically used for include 8 kg 12 kg 16, 16 kg, 24, kg 32 kg, and 24 kg. The kettlebell has gained popularity in recent decades, it is possible to find many weights between these numbers readily available. As someone who's used the kettlebell for a long time and also teaches classes regularly I can confidently declare that I've used other weights than the numbers that are standard.

There are different weight guidelines for men and women. In this particular book we will focus on males. When it comes to weight training, it's best to start with by lifting light. For Kettlebells however, it's best to choose the weight that is slightly more heavy than what you think you'll manage. This will let you develop your technique and strength without growing beyond your initial size too fast. Be cautious when using the weight and stick to what you're comfortable doing. One of the last things I would like is for you to be injured due to moving up too quickly.

The general consensus is that I advise novices to start with weights ranging from 8 and 16 kilograms. Take a look and feel what you experience. If you're experienced in lifting weights but feel that you are able to handle more than the standard weights that weigh 20 or 24 kilograms instead. Check yourself and note what you're feeling. You are better informed than anyone else. There isn't a scientific formula to this. One aspect to be considered are the different units. If you are not acquainted with kilograms, you can multiply the amount by 2.2 and you'll get your weight as pounds. For instance, 8 kg multiplied by 2.2 will be 17.6 pounds.

Many people like to consider kettlebells lifting similar to dumbbell lifting. Kettlebells aren't dumbbells, however. While lifting a particular weight might be too much for dumbbell exercises, kettlebell workouts require a completely different approach. With dumbbells, you isolated certain muscles. For instance, when you curl you're primarily focused on the biceps, and only employing that muscle in the largest part. This means that you are able to lift smaller weights. When you do kettlebell exercises, such as swings, snatches, or cleans, you'll be using several muscles. This way the heavier weights are more manageable due to the increased support. This is similar to several people lifting a couch, instead of only the one or two. In the case of the exercises mentioned above you'll be using your whole upper body, your legs to provide strength and your core muscles to keep you from becoming twisted.

The most significant issue that is often neglected is that of the handle on the kettlebell. It's an integral component of the device since it's what you're holding to for the majority of your workouts. However, many people don't think about this issue. The worst thing you could have to happen is that you get a blistered, bloody hand due to an unintentional design flaw. If you repeat a lot of repetitions using a poorly-designed handle, that's precisely what you'll get. When using dumbbells, the bar is not moving too much therefore this isn't an important factor to think about. With kettlebells your hands will be moving in a circular motion, sliding back and forth and moving side-to-side continuously. If the handles are rough edges you will find your hands hating them by the end of your first exercise.

A lot of people wear gloves to provide extra protection. This is certainly an option but it could hinder the way you work. It's best to be extra attentive to the handle, so that you don't face any issues at the start. Check the handle all around including the underneath. Check that it's smooth and free of any rough edges. The handle could cause discomfort, but in the end you'll develop callouses.

The handle should be the proper size and thickness to allow for the proper gripping. It should also have sufficient distance between it and the bell. If this space is tiny, your fingers are likely to graze the bell continuously which can cause skin irritation and lead to more blisters and cuts. This can result in serious hand injuries. There's a balance to be found in this article. The handle needs to be sanded with a smooth surface, however not overly smooth, or else you'll have a weak grip. This is especially the case after a few reps, when your hands begin getting sweaty. It's not ideal your kettlebell to fall off your fingers. You can also wear gloves, however it is better to stay clear of gloves if you can.

I understand that many people are looking for savings. I don't think you're going to want to put aside your entire savings to purchase kettlebells. But an item of high-quality is vital in this case. A low-cost kettlebell is likely to have an handle that is not than the best and will cause many of the problems we're trying to avoid. Additionally, kettlebells that are less expensive are prone to chipping due to the paint they typically have around them and are constructed of inferior materials as well. The plastic covers around vinyl bells can also wear away and begin to crack before you even realize it.

If you're planning to buy a kettlebell, it is best to buy the one made of cast iron as soon as possible. It will last an extended time and cost less due to less wear and wear. You'll need to purchase kettlebells that are new more frequently. A kettlebell is going to cost between 50 and 300 dollars. Find the cheapest kettlebell that you can afford and still offers value for money however, you should never compromise quality to get the cost. There's no point in purchasing a kettlebell in the present just because it's less expensive, only to have to purchase a new kettlebell just a few weeks later in the future due to the fact that you didn't choose wisely initially.

Be sure to consider your individual comfort. It's not worth spending some money when the kettlebell you purchase is causing injuries or just isn't comfortable for you. Think about your objectives and then make your choice with care. It can help you avoid discomfort, heartache and money in the end. Here are some additional aspects to consider when purchasing kettlebells.

There should be some level at the base or at the at the bottom part of the bell. Avoid bells with a base that's entirely round as it will cause lots of discomfort when doing certain exercises.

Alongside the outer part of the kettlebell breaking down, kettlebells that have vinyl covers can also become extremely slippery. When your hands become slippery, the likelihood of sustaining a serious injury increases dramatically. Imagine a kettlebell falling out of your hands and falling on your feet or striking another person. It's not a pleasant sight.

Make sure you research reliable brands. A reputable kettlebell manufacturer will offer anti-rust and antichip protection. This indicates they are sure of their brand and are willing to provide the promise. If a specific manufacturer is unable to assure this, they're likely to choose the wrong type of material. Again, don't cut corners to get a better manufacturer. Most likely, you'll pay more for the product and placing your security at risk.

How flexible do you intend to be? If you're looking to incorporate as many different exercises as you can, think about purchasing a variety of kettlebells that have various weights.

I know how online purchasing is a huge market in the present. I'm not knocking it. I like the fact to be able to have items delivered to their homes even if they are unable to locate them in shops. I'd suggest against buying kettlebells on the internet until you know what you're searching for. If you are buying kettlebells for the first time I would suggest shopping in person to ensure you gain a feel for the kettlebell. If the gym in your area offers kettlebells, test the kettlebells out and see if you feel about the idea. Be aware that it's an investment, so it is important to ensure that you're well-informed.

After you've purchased the kettlebell for your first time, it is all set to roll. Set yourself up for a workout that you've never experienced before. You'll be amazed the benefits that a single piece of equipment could bring.

ADVICE SUR HAND PROTECTION

If you've ever done exercise of any kind you know the possibility of harming your hands in the course of time. It's likely to happen to some extent, however there are many ways that you can reduce the risk. Believe me, my fellow men when I say to you that you don't need to live with dry cracks painful, and hand-scarred hands if they do not wish to. I know I believe it's an indication of strength, I suppose. But, I'd rather leave my hands unattended to use them later on.

We've already given you some suggestions on how to choose the right handle. Here are some more useful (pun intended) ways to protect your hands, which you can apply daily. It is difficult to be aware of how vital the hands of your are till you're no more able to use them. We should avoid the hands at the gym, will we? Contrary to gloves, these methods won't affect the duration of your workout or your performance. These are easy routines that you can follow during the day.

Moisturize Daily:

Be careful not to do this near to your workout time, so that your hands do not become slippery. There's no shame, gentlemen, when you moisturise your hands. The ideal time to do this is after your hands have been cleaned for example, after showering. Make sure to moisturize twice a day with an excellent moisturizer or lotion. Apply this treatment at the beginning of the day and at night before going to go to bed. This is the best method to prevent cracked, dry hands. Whatever way you push that kettlebell, you'll be confident shaking the hands of someone else.

Make sure to wash your hands daily:

This is a great exercise regardless of whether you have hands that have been trained or you are trying to avoid them. It's a great way to maintain your hands' softness. Warm your hands with warm water for around 15 minutes every day. It is possible to add Epsom salt into the water to achieve more effective outcomes. After the soak, you can use what's known as a pumice rock or a filer to gradually scrape off the rough areas on your hands. This can help rid your hands of any hard, scaly skin, such as calluses which have formed from exercising. It will also keep your hands perfectly smooth and soft regardless of how much you train and toss the kettlebell around.

Beware of picking at calluses:

It's tempting to get your hands on calluses and attempt to remove them. The majority of men would love to do this. But, it will make things worse for you. Every occasion you repeat this procedure, your skin will get more robust and thicker. Calluses that are a few inches long can cause discomfort and be visually unpleasant. If you are interested, you can refer to the previous two interventions I talked about.

Although men are conscious of how they look, men also think about looking good. Some of these actions might not look masculine to some, but I assure you that paying focus on how you appear isn't un-manly. The greatest men of the past were concerned about their appearance. The famous Frank Sinatra would get manicures often, and nobody would ever dare to consider him an homme. Also, if you're concerned about the people who laugh on your hand, show them a solid grip you learn during kettlebell exercises. The laughter will cease quickly.

A FEW OTHER CONSIDERATIONS:

Similar to any other exercise equipment and routines, you must be aware of some things to consider. I recommend getting a proper medical check-up before beginning any new exercise program. There could be contraindications to you to use the kettlebell, and you must be aware of before beginning. If you do not take these precautions, it could cause grave problems for you.

The first thing to do is look at your medical background. Are there any medical conditions like heart disease or diabetes, that might prevent you from lifting kettlebells? Are there joint or other conditions that you should consider. Take a moment to think about these aspects before you dive into this book.

What was your training history? Are you a fitness nut or more of a couch-surfer? Be aware of your fitness level prior to engaging in these exercises. Of course, we'll begin from scratch and everyone must learn the fundamentals first.

In the end, what kind of area do you possess? If you are training for kettlebells you'll need plenty of space to move around and swing the bell. If you aren't able to fit it at home, you might have locate a new place to move to. The device is simple to move about so that shouldn't be a problem. You can carry it anyplace. Also, think about your shoes. It is advised to walk barefoot, however when you do have to put on shoes, select ones that aren't overly cushioned. Shoes for weightlifting over running are suggested.

Chapter 6: Warm-Up and Cool Down

Cool down and warm up

It is essential to warm up prior to beginning any excise exercise and kettlebell training isn't an one's only choice. You must warm up correctly to avoid injury to muscles. Mobility is crucial for any workout. Moving your joints allows for mobility without compensating while reducing the chance of injury. Your joints remain strong and healthy. A well-planned warm-up program will not just prepare you physically, but as well mentally and neurologically, since your body must be prepared to go into actions.

The joints that you should be focusing on are

The cervical vertebrae – neck

Shoulders - both shoulder capsules as well as the girdle

The upper back and Thoracic spine

Elbows and wrists

Upper pelvis

Lower pelvis

The ankles and knees

While a lot of warm-up exercises promote circulation and joint preparation , they focus more on the level of engagement needed for kettlebells to be moved efficiently and effectively.

Around the globe

This is accomplished by picking the kettlebell , then the kettlebell along your waist. It is important to move the kettlebell in a smooth manner and make sure that your waistline is strong. Perform this exercise using the smallest amount of weight to ensure an effortless movement of the kettlebell across the floor and still maintain the control.

Keep an arc around the kettlebell and don't swing the kettlebell low in front and back. The midline should be steady with a minimum deviation from the upright position. The focus of the workout should be on improving control and mastery at lifting the kettlebell in space. Don't move your weight to adjust the movement that the kettlebell follows. The kettlebell shouldn't wander off course while it is moving through your hands. Because your body is smart enough to determine which direction feels natural and comfortable, you must always strive to keep a healthy balance with your dominant side and non dominant side.

Figure eight

It requires a sturdy and stationary body, and the only movement you can do is the arms and kettlebell. This exercise warms your hip hinge and legs. Start with the wide stance, and then smoothly move it between the legs. You then move it around one leg and then back to the opposite leg, drawing the figure eight.

Halos

It allows you to adjust and move the kettlebell, while keeping a solid and stable midline. It provides a full

Chapter 7: Advanced Exercises

Advanced routines are intended for those looking for harder kettlebell exercise. Make sure you are safe when you are doing your exercise.

Alternating renegade row

The main target is the middle back

Put two kettlebells on your floor with your feet separated. Put your hands and toes on the floor in a plank. Your body should remain straight and extended. Utilize the kettlebells to provide assistance for the upper part of your body. Pull one kettlebell towards the floor, while rowing the kettlebell in the opposite direction. Take your shoulder blade in a slack position and flex your elbows , pulling it towards your side. Lower the kettlebell down to the floor. Switch the kettlebell over to the other hand. Repeat this several times.

Double Kettlebell Alternating Hang Clean

Goals: hamstrings and forearms, biceps

Keep your feet separated. Set two kettlebells ahead of you. Start to get into this position starting by pulling your body back, while keep your head straight. Make sure you clean one kettlebell from your shoulders, while holding on one kettlebell to another. Then, quickly drop the upper kettlebell, while lifting the kettlebell on the bottom up. Perform as many repetitions in the time allotted.

Push-ups using kettlebells

The main targets are chest and shoulders.

Set the kettlebell onto the ground. In a plank, you can drop down with your feet on the floor. Place one hand on the floor , while another is clinging your kettlebell. Keep your elbows extended. Then begin to drop your body to the lowest point you can while maintaining your straight back. You can quickly reverse your movements as you push the kettlebell to the side. Switch hands as you move. Keep moving and repeat the process in a circular motion.

Open kettlebells with clean hands.

Goals: Hamstrings, glutes and lower back.

Set the kettlebell onto the ground. Take it by the handle and then pull it up by stretching your arms and then moving it between your hips and legs. Lift the kettlebell towards your shoulders. The kettlebell should be released towards the front and grab the handle using both hands. Lower the kettlebell, and repeat the motion.

One kettlebell's arm split, and snatch

Goals: shoulders, hamstringsand quadriceps

Place one kettlebell in your hand and then squat. Reverse the motion quickly while extending your knees and hips. The kettlebell should be raised over your head. After you've extended your body, you can lower into an upright position, as you push the kettlebell up over your head. One leg should be forward, and the other leg behind. Make sure you move your hips forward and then lock the kettlebell above your head with the same fluid movement. Sit up and hold the kettlebell in your head. Your feet should be together, then lower the kettlebell.

Kettlebell pistol Squat

The goals are quadriceps, calves, and quadriceps.

The kettlebell should be held by the horns by using two hands. Take one leg off the floor and squat another leg. Squat down and bend the knee while being seated. Put the kettlebell on top of your. Take a break for a few seconds and then reverse the motion by keeping your chest and head straight. Lower your body, and repeat the movement.

Bent press

Goals: abdominals, hamstrings and lower back and shoulders

Cleanse the kettlebell by transferring it through your hips and legs. Bring it up towards your shoulders and turn your wrists while you move. Then, lean towards the opposite side of your kettlebell. Continue until you're in a position to touch the ground using your free hand. Be sure to keep your eye at the kettlebell. Make sure to press the weight vertically with your elbows while keeping your body parallel towards the floor. The kettlebell should be placed in front of your head. Bring the kettlebell over your shoulder , and repeat the motion a few times.

Chapter 8: Kettlebell Fat Loss Workout

The program has been made for those with a primary objective to shed the most fat off their body. it incorporates light weight methods, high reps, and other techniques to achieve this goal.

The tools of trade needed to complete this exercise will include:

For women 8 kg kettlebells

For males - 16 kg kettlebells

The weights are suitable for an individual who is just beginning their journey and an intermediate.

A 5-kg medicine ball is available , you can make use of a set of weight plate or water bottle.

An open area in order that if you happen to fall the bell it will not cause structural damage that is serious.

The Workout

It is necessary do the exercise four to five times and train at least twice a week. The most effective number of iterations each week are 3-4. The workouts are in the following order:

Double handed kettlebell swings 15 reps:

The guidelines are identical to those provided in the previous chapter.

Clean 12 - 15 reps each arm:

The entire idea behind this exercise is to quickly raise a kettlebell behind your shoulders before placing it on the high point on your upper forearms. Then, you can do either kettlebell presses or front squats. It is important to note that unlike the barbell clean kettlebell clean is required for many other exercises , but is not a complete exercise on its own.

However, the exercise targets certain muscle groups which include the glutes, hamstrings core and lower back.

Begin by taking the deadlift posture, putting the kettlebell between your legs using the right side of your hand. Clean is a quick motion on its own. in reality, you're supposed to be doing an upwards jump at the same time, however the kettlebell absorbs this energy and turns it into something far easier to manage.

The kettlebell is pushed up, however instead of having the arms fully extended move them back a bit to make sure the weight is closer to your body. This also stops the muscles of the arms from being overused. Consider them as ropes that shift weights from one spot from one position to the other.

Once the kettlebell has reached chest height, you can quickly slide your arms beneath the bell until the kettlebell comes to a complete stop and the position is locked.

You'll now be in the clean or racked posture. Take note of how your wrists are straight, and your forearms and hands are slender.

Tips for power - before you learn the correct technique first, you need to master what to do when you lower your kettlebell away from the rack position. This is done using the kettlebell placed in the rack, retaining the rack position using one arm while using the other to lift the kettlebell with the gripping hand. After that, lowering the weight to the deadlift position will do the trick. You'll need repeat these steps several of times before mastering it, but once master it, you'll have no difficulty performing the exercise correctly.

Press 12 - 15 reps each arm:

Kettlebell presses are an effective exercise that works the shoulder, laterals and the biceps. For the exercise to be performed it is necessary to first take the rack position, following the instructions mentioned above.

Begin in the rack with your body tight, shoulders down, and elbows in a tucked-in position. Make sure your laterals are to the sides and strengthen your abdominal muscles to ensure that your waist is able to provide adequate support to keep your position. Avoid trying to lift the kettlebell uphill by drawing strength via your legs.

From the rack, start turning your shoulders to the side until your forearms are horizontal and the rear of your hand that is carrying the load is in front of you.

When pressing a kettlebell, the bell should follow a banana-shaped curve when raised outwards, and then back up. Also, make sure to squeeze into your arms as you lift it in the vertical position the next step.

Finally, pull the kettlebell straight up to get the full arm lockdown while you go about it.

Here are some suggestions to help you get started on the best kettlebell press

When you are in the rack position lower your shoulders as far as you can to ensure that the muscles between the shoulders have been stretched. This will allow the muscles to be loaded and gain more leverage. the elbows need to be in contact with hipbones in the stretch position.

Flex the rear muscles (laterals) to make them diverge. This will enable the body to attain greater stability, which will aid in your vertical lifting.

Grab the handles as tightly as you can. This will not only enable you to have more control of the bell, but aid in engaging your arms when you lift.

When pressing the kettlebell, concentrate on your shoulders and the laterals. Always draw strength from these muscles, not from the biceps.

In lieu of thinking about lifting the kettlebell, concentrate on removing yourself of the kettlebell.

Russian twist 8 reps per side:

The task is quite simple and requires only a little of preparation beforehand.

Place your feet on the ground and then sit up in a seated position with a kettlebell at your side.

Make sure your legs are slightly bent.

Place the kettlebell on your side, and then pick it up.

Make a twisting motion to ensure that the kettlebell is on the opposite side of your body.

You should go as far back as you can during the turn, so long as you're avoiding the back.

Be in control of the action and make sure you do it in a controlled manner.

Push press 12 - 15 reps on each side:

Start the workout in the push-up position. your body needs to be in a plank. Stand facing the floor with both arms forming an angle vertical off the floor. However, instead of letting your hands rest upon the ground, you can grab a set of kettlebells and place your weight on the top of them.

Reduce your body as you go, while balancing on kettlebells. Get the chest to to the ground as is possible, and then moving away.

When you are in the highest spot, raise one kettlebell at a time and then place you bodyweight on kettlebell that is resting. Put your elbow behind your back and place the wrist placed as near to the abdominal area as you can.

Lower the weight you lifted back to its original position and then perform a second lift, this time using the opposite shoulder.

A single leg: 15 reps of RDL on each side:

Keep your posture straight and keep your feet spread shoulder width and then grab the kettlebell using your left hand.

Start to raise your left leg and while doing so then lower the rest your body in a direction of the forward movement so that your balance remains.

Continue to lower yourself back to a comfortable level until the kettlebell barely touches the ground. Then you can lift yourself up again.

Repetitions of Windmills 12 times each side:

This exercise is an excellent option to increase strength in the upper part of your body. It targets the oblique, laterals, shoulders and the core. It's more of a strengthening exercise, and the most effective method of learning the technique is to start by working with lighter weights.

Standing shoulder width apart, keep your feet pointed outwards.

Hold the kettlebell with your right hand and lift it up vertically. Continue moving until your arm is locked and then kick your left hip to ensure you don't fall over. Left hand must be in a neutral position and should be set free.

Breathe in and keep your abdominal muscles in a tight position while you perform the vertical pull. This will stop any sudden jerks from damaging your back.

The kettlebell is in your sight. move it to the left hip. Move your left hand and put it on the left thigh. As you push the kettlebell downwards, you can lean the left leg bit, but remember that the leg should remain locked.

Keep bending your hips, then slide your left hand through the thigh and lower leg until you are on the floor. If you aren't able to achieve the flexibility required, simply lower your leg as far as you can. In time, your flexibility will improve so that you'll be in a position do this in a way that is effective.

Do this by squeezing your glutes. go all the up.

Repeat the process with the other hand.

If you're having difficult times doing this exercise, then test it out without adding any weight until you attain your optimal range of motion.

When you are doing the exercise, be sure that you do not do a backward bend. It is also essential to maintain full control during the workout. many people have injured their oblique muscles by lifting the kettlebell vertically before dropping the kettlebell on their head and aggravated the injury.

The Routine:

The following routine is packed with an entire week of workout. the goal is to repeat the exercise three times per week for six weeks. The tables serve as a guideline , and will aid in tracking your progress after the completion of every week.

When you're doing the exercises, try to do the smallest number of reps to be in a position to breathe every now and then. It is permitted to rest for 1 - 2 minutes between each round , but you don't have to do every single round, 3-4 would be well.

As numerous rounds as you can within 20 minutes.

Start and finish each circuit with five minutes on the treadmill and stationary bikes.

Monday's Workout

Weight Rd. 1 Rd. 2 Rd. 3 Rd. 4 Rd. 5 Rd. 6

Double kettlebell swing

Clean

Press

Russian twist

Press down

Single leg RDL

Windmills

Wednesday's Workout

Weight Rd. 1 Rd. 2 Rd. 3 Rd. 4 Rd. 5 Rd. 6

Double kettlebell swing

Clean

Press

Russian twist

Press down

Single leg RDL

Windmills

Workout on Friday

Weight Rd. 1 Rd. 2 Rd. 3 Rd. 4 Rd. 5 Rd. 6

Double kettlebell swing

Clean

Press

Russian twist

Press down

Single leg RDL

Windmills

Chapter 9: How to and Don'ts to Kettlebell Benefits

We live in a vast universe of information that is endless, but we occasionally look at the risks of this technological advancement. Innovation has helped us travel across oceans at the blink of our eyes.

There are many ways to use a kettlebell.

Perhaps not as many, but in the present of collaboration and shaping the kettlebell into an essential training tool for teachers and students.

With all the information (and lies) available in relation to the chime's sound, it's easy to get lost.

For people who are just beginning, and even more surprising for those who have accumulated years of experience This quick guide will guide you along the way.

Here are five rules and don'ts of your kettlebell to protect you from soaring gains.

The 5 Don'ts to Avoid for Kettlebell Benefits

It is time to move the kettlebells away from these. So far as I am able to see, in the the many years of using kettlebells, the five main points are the main factors that hinder people in the direction of getting the most from the kettlebell.

1. Be careful not to take it To The Limit

Naturally If something is acceptable there are a few people out there who believe that many more ought to be better. If an action is considered acceptable and we can raise it. If the grab is accepted then we can do it over the course of 60 minutes.

If you don't plan to compete in kettlebell sports There's no reason to push your kettlebell training to its limits. In the best case scenario, you'll be exhausted, and in the worst case scenario, you'll create a physical problem. The ability to maintain equilibrium is essential. This is true for pretty much everything in everyday life too.

If you're new to kettlebells and want to get started with one foot, then three complete body exercises that target every week's development plan is an excellent deal.

2. Make sure not to go Too Light

The usual fitness centers and retail chains all over the world will let you agree that a kettlebell that weighs 10lbs is everything men's needs, and 5lbs is more than enough for a woman.

If you're thinking about it, old friend, I'd rather not to blow your pot bubble, but should you want to see any benefits from the chime, then you'll need to push yourself.

Naturally, we collectively must begin somewhere, and perhaps it is the best burden for you. The majority of the times (a number I've just came up with to make an argument, and is not yet not certain to be accurate) students tend to be light. If you're one of the people who do, you're fine.

There's still a lot to be expected. There's no standard to follow since each person is unique. However, here's a useful guide to healthy, non-injured individuals:

Ladies: 4kg-12kg

Men: 12kg-20kg

If you're fairly solid and fit , then you should be aiming towards the higher quality of the range. If you feel that a lot don't appeal to you take a step back.

There are exceptions, and regardless of whether you are able to deadlift 40kg, it's best to choose a kettlebell can be used for a variety of exercises using instead of just one to get the highest benefits.

3. Be careful not to go too Overweight

On the other hand, being excessively heavy won't help in the same way. If you're able to stretch your self-image and flexing your muscles, you'll be able to do more damage than any other thing. Because you've seen it on the internet or in one of the "games" isn't a guarantee that you're ready.

The importance of testing yourself is paramount but when you're breaking the framework for the reasons behind lifting a particular weight, the risk of dangers are greater than anything you could be doing.

Most injuries are caused by the breakdown of the first or the other burden or exhaustion. The weight of heavyweight is essential to develop endurance in the event that you stay within your limits. It's not difficult to establish an aim of pushing at a heavier or more weight, and even becoming exuberant.

If you're using the weight or not, you can work within a certain rep range. You can stop the set once structure breaks down, and even more surprising an additional set or two prior to the set.

4. Be careful not to exceed Your Limits

The fact that you must accomplish something doesn't mean you're able to complete something. Will is important, but the capability is vital.

If I had a nickel every time I've witnessed someone performing a specific move such as the grab in a normal rec center, with no details about the process other than watching a short video, I'd be an incredibly rich man.

Locating a trusted trainer in your neighborhood or recording informative sessions will benefit your body. Web-based media is an extremely risky option in the event that you're not a kettlebell expert. Moving, amazing innovations, or projects that have an enormous volume could look attractive, however, in the event that you're unprepared for it , take a step back.

Check where you stand with your current scope of action on an individual development plan. Understanding where you stand will provide you with a good understanding of what direction to take. Check out the channel Durability available on Onnit Academy On Demand to explore the surrounding areas and to open new areas for development.

5. Don't think that the Kettlebell Is Only For Cardio

It is usually effective with people who are strong and also rodents from the rec center. In contrast to a deadlift of 500 pounds, even the largest kettlebell would not possibly be compared. It is evident that it can be thought of as a cardio device. You should do some ballistic movement towards the end of your exercise and then kick out, correct?

Yes, dear old friend you'll miss the benefits of strength that come from the incredible kettlebell routine. Double kettlebell work, massive one-arm swings, bowed presses, flagon squats and amazing streams will definitely do more than send your heart pumping. It's all about paying being aware of what's possible.

A great program to build great fortitude and strength is to use kettlebells (or two) to build a circuit with strength. Select 3-5 exercises using a weight that will be 5 to 8 RM for each development. Each development should be performed for 5 reps, resting a time between sets out.

You can, for instance, perform the flagon squat, press as well as a rebel column and one-arm swing. Another fantastic way to integrate your ringer with the strength-training session is by using the idea of developing the OTM (on at the time) type of meeting.

This will give you plenty of volume and keeps reps at a low. My top recommendation is the spotless double front squat that can be set for groups of 3-6 for 8-12 sets. This will give you plenty of room for growth because you are unable to alter the weights without a problem.

We've already covered that, these are the must-knows to get the most benefit possible from kettlebell training.

The 5 Things to Do for Kettlebell Benefits

1. Do not use the kettlebell to Strengthen Weaknesses

Shortcomings. We all have them , and we're prone to grabbing them tightly for the sake of our lives. They can be an excuse to attempt more difficult changes. The chime may help you in getting rid of those insular, fixed focus points that keep you from progressing.

Between clothes, arm bars, windmills, and alcoholics presses kettlebells are awe-inspiring strength but also a remarkable range of motion from your hips up to your shoulders, as well as everything in the middle.

For a while I've told potential customers "probably the most beneficial feature of the kettlebell is that it makes you comfortable uncomfortable positions." This is a great way to build evidence of injuries for customers and competitors.

It is possible to consolidate your testing skills as a warm-up or I choose the ones that are the most difficult based on my body's abilities and then spend the whole time playing with the exercises.

In this case, I'll combine an extended warm-up and then hit various sets (never to disappoint) of presses, lushes and deep challis squats using lighter weights. Although these workouts aren't necessarily the most challenging because of weight or strength however, they test.

However, if you do not make use of them in testing simply by adding one of one of the most important developments (the swing) and you'll increase the hamstring's adaptability, which makes it more versatile, robust. Because of the position of the kettlebell even squeeze it will pull your arm back a bit more stretching your lats while open your shoulders slightly.

2. Do Make Use of Them to Create an energizing backside

How can a better stable posterior means? It's basically everything is bouncing higher and higher, running faster while kicking with more intensity and more stable posture. The hamstrings and glutes of your legs are the best place to focus your force for increasing hip speed and dangerous fortitude.

Every muscle that is in your spine chain gets strengthened by ballistic kettlebell advancements. This will separate them away from the free-weights. Yes, you can do free weight cleans, presses, squats and columns, but high repetition ballistic handweight work isn't so easy to perform.

What makes the posterior stronger is that it performs ballistic work using a the pivot (bowing to the hips) by this method, putting more power in the back.

The solution? Swings (or various variations of them) performed at least three times per week. It can be done with lighter and heavier weights and the focus should be on 50 to 200 repetitions (not necessarily immediately).

Sets can be split and performed in a stepping stool fashion at any time or paired with a fitness routine such as pushups to make it a more vigorous gathering.

3. Do not use kettlebells to build an Iron Grip

A strong hold is more effective than what the wellness industry credits it with. While it's not quite so hot as lean abs it's not just for arm-grapplers and farmers of cows.

The off-kilter configuration of the ringer provides the kettlebell an advantage over other devices because it entails the lower arm flexed in the rack as well as the in the overhead position. Combine that with the kettlebell's streams, shuffling and ballistic advancements to strengthen your grip at every place.

In the meantime, try simple circuits and structures that don't place the weight down. It will allow you to hold massively when you're done with enough weight. Concentrate on circuits that last at least 60 seconds and with the weight you are able to deal without having to put down.

In the end, try higher-level schedules and shuffling the walls to let go of the force that the bell.

4. Do Use Kettlebells To Train In Different Planes

A substantial portion of exercise for solidarity is completed with the trunk being flexed and then augmented with an occasional rotational development ball toss. The greatest strength of the ringer lies in its ability to switch between different development perfectly, which includes developments which take you away from the plane of sagittal.

Deadlifts and squats are both amazing however, when you mix amazing developments using any form of sidelong punches and 360 grabs, you'll build the ability to fortify yourself from a multitude of different points.

The force moving (what we've dubbed the new argument along with kettlebell running) is essentially reflective. There aren't any standardizations. There are no sets or reps. It's just a matter of moving and it allows you to study various areas of motion, planes and design concepts for development.

Set the clock to two minutes using an object that you can work with throughout the course of every phase of development. After that, join all development, combine the work of rotation, and then explore it.

5. Do Use Kettlebells To Simplify Your Training Life

If you're a coach or a class leader, kettlebells can be a great way to guide clients through an array of new developments that can provide the strength and shape in record time. If you're an individual expert, nothing can beat the simplicity of a few the chimes or some outside air.

It's not difficult to get involved in the "more is more" attitude with regard to equipment used in exercise centers in normal locations. Hand weights, racks as well as link machines and stomach muscles stations, and the list goes on.

A few kettlebells allow you to include dynamic movements to your daily routine of exercises, allowing you to reduce. A break in the top down, speed driven schedules could be an impressive change in speed.

A few simple edifices and innovations can assist you in advancing your solidarity journey without skipping an itch and without the enormous amounts of equipment and weight that are required.

An easy way to do this is to limit your tools to a kettlebell and mace or club, as well as suspension coaches and your body for an advanced physique without the puff.

Which is more effective? Dumbbells or Kettlebells?

Visit any fitness center and you'll see two types of free equipment that are the traditional hand weights and the newest addition, kettlebells. Both have benefits and enthusiasts, but the same question is asked frequently when it comes to seeing results, should one claim that one is better than the other compared to the other? Experts have a few suggestions about what to select and when to choose.

Visit any fitness center where you'll find two types of free equipment such as the hand weights and the newest kettlebells. Both have benefits and fans, but the same question is asked frequently in getting results, should you say that one is superior over the other? In this case, experts have an opinion about what to select and when to choose.

Dynamic Moving: Kettlebells

In terms of touchy changes, real changes, kettlebells are the ideal. If you're aiming to lift weights or plyo enhancements or in the event that you're participating in a sport that demands instability (like B-ball and CrossFit games) studies suggest that kettlebells can lead to greater gains.Trusted Source

Select these exercises for routines that include a number of major muscle groups, and also include performing the movements in a important way. The most common kettlebell movements are cleans, grabs, windsmills Turkish clothing, and most importantly, the swing of the kettlebell.

The swings are also unique due to the fact that they can boost your heart rate, providing the cardiovascular system as well as strengthening benefits as stated by Dell Polanco, lead trainer at BRICK New York. As opposed to a basic twist or press, a kettlebell swing is a powerful force that activates your entire back chain of muscles including your glutes, hamstrings and the erector spinae (back muscles) He explains.

Essential Movements: Dumbbells

"Free weights are amazing for an ounce in everything" says Nikki Reifschneider as the associate supervisor of personal training and wellness in the University of Miami. "You could start by doing important exercises such as the chest press, shoulder press, line or squats that are hand-weighted that are held by your shoulders." The advantage is that you don't have to swing the weight around (as you do with the swing or grab) and you can make the movements more clearly, Reifschneider says.

Making Your Workout More Fun: Kettlebells

"In the event that you're bored of doing hikers or burpees Try kettlebells as part of an exercise that is HIIT," says Liz Barnet the confirmed coach of Uplift Studios in New York City. Barnet states that it's not difficult to incorporate kettlebells with an exercise finishing routine, for example, 30-

60 minutes of full-scale exertion moves to finish off.

Beginners: Dumbbells

Use hand weights only in the case of guidance from kettlebells Barnet says. In fact, all of the professionals we spoke with emphasized that hand weights are the best choice to train with weights unless you've specifically worked with a fitness trainer for kettlebells.

Enhancing grip strength: Kettlebells

Because the Horn (handle) that is the handle of the kettlebell can be larger than the freeweight, kettlebells could be ideal for enhancing the strength of your grasp, Barnet says. "For instance, a twist around the line of a kettlebell will strengthen the grip and prepare you for testing exercises like draw upwards" Barnet says.

General Fitness Dumbbells

One study revealed that, in contrast to energetic kettlebell movements important weightlifting exercises (think power cleans as well as squats) resulted in more significant improvements in strength and strength over a six-week period.Trusted Source for all, if your goal is overall health and fitness it's fine sticking to free weights. There's probably no advantage to using kettlebells.

An Extra Challenge to be added: Kettlebells

"Kettlebells have the primary point of gravity about six to eight inches away from your hand, however hand weights provide more stability," Reifschneider says. This makes actions such as kettlebell presses that are bottoms-up very challenging, as you're trying lifting the weight and then balance it so that the chime does not overturn and impact your arm. Teachers also like kettlebells because of their insecurity. They're just like the unbalanced items that you see every day. But, when added to that examination, kettlebells could be the impression of a threat and, if you're just beginning to work out, you should stick with hand weights.

Intensifying Weight Gain: Dumbbells

It's not hard to make your workouts more challenging by using an hand weight. "You do not need to use hand weights for sluggish separate push-press movement," Polanco says. "You can do hang cleans and squat cleans. These are dangerous developments." Polanco also suggests to practice a few of these dangerous movements initially using free weights before you move towards kettlebells. Remember "somewhat that a weight is something that weighs," Reifschneider says. "With every piece of equipment you could do an exercise test. It's all about your creativity."

Additionally, kettlebells don't typically have small size increases as hand weights do, Polanco says. Although a variety of companies make kettlebells with different weights dependent on the type of exercise facility has available and available, it could be difficult to find an "wonderful fitting." However the majority of fitness centers put free weights in five-pound increments, making them perfect for gaining weight step-by-step.

The Takeaway

So which one is superior? It all depends on. Anyone who is just starting out and wants to develop their strength in the fitness center must go to the free weight rack while CrossFitters and those who are performing dangerous exercises should grab kettlebells. Choose the weight that is compatible with your exercise strategy and health level and do not hesitate to decide whether you should consult an expert mentor to get an individual evaluation should there are any questions.

Chapter 10: Kettlebell Sport Vs. Kettlebell Fitness

They are two completely different worlds, so let's look at these two separately before looking at the potential benefits that could be derived from kettlebell users in general who train the method of sport.

Kettlebell fitness is something you'll find with the majority of trainers and customers. They are used to activate of multiple muscle groups and, in most cases, some kind of ballistic movement for power growth and exercises for core activation. They can be incorporated into a routine that is timed depending on the need or be used on their own for workouts that are intense. Be aware that the purpose is the primary factor in the workout.

Kettlebell sports are not for the faint of heart. Although it is possible to train in a casual manner to gain a better appreciation of what's involved but true kettlebell sports requires you to go all out to achieve a new personal best for 10 minutes without time for rest. A small proportion of people choose this path because of how challenging it can be. It isn't a stroll in the park, it's very demanding and extremely painful. If you look at the way you compare to other elite athletes, and how you compare against the world's top kettlebell lifters, you'll be able to see just how large the gap. Elite sprinters can cover 100m in under 10 seconds. A good trainer will be able to complete the same feat in about 15 seconds, if not more. While you're far from Olympic standards, you have a the ability to measure the distance between your performance and theirs. In essence, they're 50 percent more efficient than you. It is the same for numerous other sports where athletes can lift weights two or 3 times as heavy as you are able to, or leap twice as high as you. We then enter the realm of kettlebell sports where the majority of trainers will not be able to jerk a pair kettlebells that weigh 32kg. The current record in the world is 175 reps over 10 minutes. We are faced with the problem of. What is the best way to quantify the difference between something you can't do once, and something somebody else is able to do 175 times over a period of time? This is the same for the grab. Only a few trainers are able to take a 32kg kettlebell with each hand to perform reps, but world-class lifters do more than 100 reps in each hand, with no rest and with only one hand change. The distance between people who are average and elite is nearly astronomical. Because of this, the majority people who train using kettlebells will not be interested in training for the sport.

We now look at potential crossovers. Although you can't cross through a chasm in just two steps, you can certainly prepare for kettlebell sports through breaking down the exercise into smaller steps. They involve doing a certain number of exercises and then taking a break, or using an active/rest approach for a certain period of time. There are numerous benefits to kettlebell training aside from a

102

soaring endurance, mental strength and an incredible capacity for work. Modifying these intense workouts is sure to yield results that are far and beyond the results you would expect from regular sets and reps.

Standard and Competition kettlebells as well as standard cast kettlebells

The kind of kettlebell that you will use to train with may be determined by your specific training goals. If you're only planning to work out for kettlebell sports to boost your participation in long-cycle or biathlon event then competitive kettlebells that have a square handle that is made of steel should be your preferred preference. If you're considering using kettlebells to aid in losing weight and maintaining general fitness and fitness, then the two-handed swing will be a significant part of your training, as it's often not possible to grip a competitive kettlebell using both hands to swing with no compromise regarding the grip. The average hand will discover that the smaller fingers have to be wrapped around the ring fingers, and the wrists have to be separated in order to align the palms or the smaller fingers rest outside of the handles. This is why it's advised that those who are trying to shed weight and general fitness, choose the standard kettlebell made of cast iron which has handles that are slightly larger than competition steel and the more prominent curve radius allows two hands to rest more comfortably between the various parts of the handle which connect with the ball. Another issue is that it is not suitable for women who are novice athletes. A kettlebell for competition of 8kg will be roughly the same as an iron kettlebell of 40kg (but it is hollow) and it could create difficulties learning the proper moves dependent on the dimensions of the ball as well as the higher level of skill required to manage it in the motion. A kettlebell of 8kg made of cast iron is about the size of an orange, and is much less intimidating than its steel counterpart. In addition to these two reasons regarding the reasons the reasons why a kettlebell made of cast iron is preferred instead of a kettlebell for competition, the decision is entirely up to the person and the type of workout they are planning be varied, covering multiple exercises, or possibly use two kettlebells at a at the same time. Different people will inform you different things based on their experiences. People who train using kettlebells for competitions will say that you must only train with kettlebells that are competitive, while others advise using kettlebells for competition only in case you train to and participate in competitions. Do not let this put you off, just choose a method and begin moving because there are many more important aspects to think about!

Kettlebell training variables

Plan your workouts

A kettlebell routine of basic quality would always comprise of certain functional movements that prepare for the workout. They will engage muscles and joints throughout a range of motion. They should also be mapped to the exercises that are part of the exercise. The time of the workout and the demands of the athlete/client they would typically then move to joints mobility or dynamic stretching. The kettlebell workout just requires a few exercises or complexes to give the full body benefit. When you look at an average bell curve populace, 90% of people would benefit from the following exercise -

Two hand swings lasting 10 minutes, with gradual adjustments to active and rest variables, and finally the weight that is used. An example is to taking 30 seconds to swing and then take a rest for 30 seconds or beginning with 10 sets every minute.

Kettlebell exercises

The most frequently asked questions regarding kettlebells tend to fall on the three categories below

How can I come up with my routine?

Do I need to use kettlebells in conjunction in conjunction with my current workout?

Do kettlebells work as a set?

In the first question we're dealing with the design of the program and often some element of periodisation. While kettlebells can be a useful tool for training, but they're certainly not the best solution to all issues. If, for instance, the individual is in strong phase, then kettlebells are not suitable for bilateral squats however, they could be a factor in bilateral strength/stability, and could help develop better core control by utilizing certain exercises like overhead squats and lunges. One good rule of thumb to follow is to choose the correct equipment for the job. It's not a good idea to offer a beginner the strength phase of 90. On the other hand, an experienced athlete won't see any strength improvement from a kettlebell weight of 16kg beyond warming up and interval training.

When creating a routine, it is essential to think about the various variables that are involved as well as their interplay. A few general guidelines are provided below:

Training Goal The load* Reps Sets Rest

Strength +85% 1-6 2-6 2-5 2-5 minutes

Power Single repetition of 80-90% in 1-2, 3-5 2-5 minutes

Power - Multi reps 75-85% for 3-5 minutes. 2-5 minutes

Hypertrophy between 67 and 85%, 6-12 3-3 30-90 secs

Endurance - 67 percent 12+ 2-3 30 seconds

Variables in training and their interactions

The way you manipulate variables like the amount of reps, sets, load, frequency , and recovery can have the most significant influence on how efficient the training session is to meet the goal that the participant. If you don't have enough knowledge about these interactions and the way they should be altered when an athlete gains strength and develops, there is always the possibility that progress will be slow or even non-existent because the program isn't fit for the purpose. The most important thing to consider is that the capacity to work will be the primary focus at first because good movements are created with the use of a weight that is repeated several times during a session to ensure the sameness. Gradually, this will shift in volume, and greater intensities , as sufficient pressure must be put on the body in order to facilitate growth and adaptation.

Although we love our kettlebell workout however, we'll be among the first providers of training to acknowledge that they are not the solution to all problems. Kettlebells can be an efficient part of an fitness program for athletes however they're only an element of the solution. It is difficult to work to your the maximum amount of strength without access to adequate equipment such as bars, stands and cages. Although they are able to be used to supplement the needs of those who are looking to improve their fitness but the more experienced athlete will require a larger toolbox.

The Force-Velocity Curve

It is the Force-Velocity curvature (F-Vc) is one of the primary aspects to consider when designing programs. The relationship between these two components can be interpreted by following. Large loads are moved at a slower pace and lighter load can move at high speed. As an example, take the difference in time when you perform 5kg in your own personal deadlift, and hitting a tennis ball or jumping over three small obstacles in succession for the duration of. On the vertical axis,, we are able to see that the more strength, the less the time or speed. This line is the place where you work on maximum strength adaptations that are with very small reps with high intensity, as well as long recovery times in order to refill the system. As we progress across the horizontal axis of velocity and the force and load reduce, the velocity grows. Imagine how fast you'll be able to do a deadlift that's half of your maximum effort, compared to 5kg less than the maximum effort. When we are preparing for power training, the weight should be able to be moved with speed and yet at a certain percentage of intensity in order to achieve the desired effects of training. Since the basis for explosive strength is a strong foundation of strength, it is essential that strength remain maintained throughout an exercise phase because it will decline in less than 2 weeks, if it's not directly stimulated. The power can also be developed by using various drills and exercises and also require a solid base of strength before being incorporated into a routine. When you continue to move across the horizontal line the load starts to decrease into exercise equipment like medicine ball overhead throws, rebounds and cable machines that permit freedom of movement with the use of a lighter load. It is recommended that the concept that of dynamic correspondence (also called particularity) is addressed by training to guarantee that that the training meets the requirements for the particular sport. Consider it as as a pyramid, where you build solid foundations of strength across all joints and muscle groups across the entire range to minimize the risk of injury due to imbalances or weakness. Then, you incorporate power training to build explosiveness equipped to utilize the gains in strength through fast muscle contractions and greater threshold motor unit activation. The speed end will always include a variety of micro loaded and unloaded exercises that are similar to the sport and at the speeds that the sport requires. While strength is essential, but it can also be slow. The majority of professional sports are slow. Therefore, there has to be a conversion to power , and then speed. The best example of this was found in research conducted in Greece conducted by Tsimahidis and coworkers in the year 2010. They showed that a short sprinting exercise after the squats exercise was a significant influence on strength, vertical jump , and acceleration, compared to control groups for a 10-week time span.

One final thing to think about when using the F-Vc is the fact the fact that multiple aspects can be covered during the same session. If you're having all day long, warmup sets could be targeted to improve speed. This will be beneficial because you'll be refreshed prior to the beginning of the training session. If you're having a maximal Squat-day the speed squats and jump squats can be effectively added to the warmup stages. In particular, by relating the FVC to kettlebell training, you will see that only a handful of exercises are able to be altered, such as the Snatch and Jerk. The good thing is that both are strength exercises and therefore can serve as a fantastic addition to the development of working rate of force (RFD). Certain movements, like the clean and the swing are characterized by a specific timing into them as they depend on pendulum motion and if they are interrupted, it usually results in a damage to the mechanics and efficiency of the motion pattern. They will typically be taught to improve strength or endurance dependent on the factors of reps and loads and the way they are controlled.

Bioenergetics

A frequently overlooked aspect of exercise physiological physiology is the energy system that is dominant in the specific training program and the way it affects the sport and goals of an athlete. One excellent example was an unconclusive debate about the significance of VO2max for elite Taekwondo players due to it being an anaerobic and explosive sport. Although it is true that having a greater VO2 max could aid in recovery during interval after rounds, the results were obvious that an excessive emphasis on a cardio-based approach is not enough to allow an elite athlete to become as explosive as is possible over a long period of time.

Bioenergetics examines the the production of energy and its transfer within living organisms. This offers us a useful guideline for matching training plans with objectives to ensure that they are in line with. For instance, the requirement of a weightlifter who is an elite athlete to lift close to and more than their maximum weight 6 times during competition does not require a huge amount of training in VO2 max. However, it has been proven that this kind of concentrate on the wrong type of energy system can actually decrease explosive power output in the long run (Baechle and Earle 2008).

The three fundamental energy systems The three basic energy systems

Phosphagen

Glycolysis

Oxidative

The primary function of these systems of energy is to replenish muscles with adenosine triphosphate (ATP). ATP is the mammalian equivalent to petrol or diesel for cars. The table below can be an idea of which system is dominant in relation to exertion, duration and the rest/recovery rate required.

Power % at maximum energy system Energy system Exercise time Work/rest ratio

90-100 Phosphagen 5-10 seconds 1:12 - 1:20

75 to 90 Fast glycolysis between 15 and 30 second 1:3 - 1;5

30 to 75 Fast glycolysis, oxidative processes 1-3 mins 1:3 - 1;4

20-30 Oxidative more than 3 mins 1:1 - 1:3

Reproduced from Baechle as well as Earle (2008)

For instance, think about the 100-meter sprint. If you were required to put in an all-out maximal effort, and try to match or beat the personal record you have set, there's the possibility that you won't be able to replicate this event until a complete recovery has occurred and could last for more than 10-minutes (most likely and not in that date!). It's highly unlikely that this full-on effort to the phosphagen system can be repeated in less than 2 minutes, based on the demands it puts on the system as well as the amount of time required to replenish the deficiency. But, multiple sprints of 20 meters at 50-60% capacity can easily be completed one after the one with a time rest of only a few minutes. The lower the total intensity of the exercise is, the more time it will be mastered and less recuperation is needed for it to be performed with consistency. Studies have shown that 5 second sprints with a recovery time of 120 seconds do not show a reduction in performance for 15 rounds. In reality the fatigue phase only starts to impact performance after recovery is reduced to 90 seconds, and this does not occur until round 11 (Balsom and co. 1992).

Kettlebell and bioenergetics training

The table above can help in the classification of kettlebell workouts according to load intensity. It is common for people to finish an exercise with kettlebells but not know exactly how they fit into the larger scheme of things, or how they can be integrated into training programmes. The following examples will aid in integrating them.

The swing of the kettlebell is the underlying element of kettlebell instruction and in addition to enhancing the capacity to work, which is essential for developing effective forces in the saggital plane of cleaning and picking up movements, it's an exercise that can be performed as a stand-alone for beginners who are progressing. When you consider the energy systems, it must be clear that using the phosphagen system to train with swings can be challenging. For instance the weight needs to be so heavy that the technique could be compromised before the system can be effectively trained with no risk. It's also possible that training at 90% of your potential for a few reps can lead to a kettlebell you are unable to reach from the floor! On the other side of the spectrum is applicable. Although low intensity is beneficial to burn fat, there should be a limit to ensure that individuals are not doing nothing but wasting time. At a rate of 20 percent of your maximum on the swing set could result in men working out using a kettlebell that weighs less than 10 kgs. The total benefit of this kind of weight is not significant because hundreds of repetitions would have to be performed for any kind of carryover or any other variables will need to be adjusted like workout speed and time between rests. It would simply not be sensible to build a marathon-running athlete by walking for 6 months in order to get them ready for the greater demands of running. Additionally, working less than the recommended capacity will not have any relationship to the long-term results and will eat away at precious workout time which could be better used in more intense intervals.

We have two remaining systems. It is crucial to look at these systems in relation to power percentages and duration. The more work you do the longer you'll be able to keep it up for. If a man can lift an a kettlebell of 24kg and pass a five-minute test of swing, then it falls into the oxidative and glycolysis fast group , based on the time taken and output percent. To boost the intensity and make sure that the exercise can last between 15 and 30 seconds, the appropriate kettlebell needs to be chosen to build the glycolysis system that is fast according to the parameters required. This involves watching performance in relation to kettlebell weights and durations and the feedback regarding perceived exertion as well as the intensity. This will help in designing to focus on particular energy system development within programs and utilize kettlebells together with other training methods to assist in attaining the objectives of the program.

Chapter 11: Kettlebell

There's a lot you can accomplish with kettlebells. Consider the intense workouts that you believed you were missing at the fitness center: bicep curls, chest presses, triceps extension back workouts shoulders presses, trapezius exercises deadlifts, squats, deadlifts, and much more.

With just one kettlebell, one kettlebell can complete all of those exercises.

You can purchase one kettlebell and be in good shape. You'll be able to feel that your life has returned to normal, and you'll feel like you're back at the gym once more. The great thing is that kettlebells are affordable and doesn't take up much spaces . Therefore, even if you reside in a tiny house you can still make use of it for every exercise you'd like to complete.

Kettlebells are available in various weights that start at 2kg to as much as 32kg. Kettlebells with lower weights are offered at a cheaper cost, and as weights get heavier in value, so do the prices. Even with a heavy capacity, cost of kettlebells isn't too expensive when compared to barbells, dumbbells and plates for weights of kg.

You're probably wondering, "wait a minute, how do I go from a slack to a exhilarated by using a kettlebell that weighs 32kg?". In reality, if you're following my advice to only use one kettlebell, a kettlebell of 32kg is unsuitable and you'd have to be working with 20kg. That means that in order to complete all exercises, you'd be restricted to using lighter weights.

It is said that you have to weight a lot in order to grow and, to tell that's the case, I have believed that. However, I did realize that you can be jacked up and lift standard weights.

Now, you're going to be thinking "I see these giants squatting 200kg for legs, lifting a 16 kg barbells to do the bench press on their chests, deadlifting up to 250kg to the lower back, and lifting 70kg to do back workout - out. How is that possible"?

It's possible, in fact. Here's why:

All it boils down to is your technique and form.

After every rep, a good method is to squeeze the appropriate muscle group, hold it for two seconds, then finish the rep with a gentle pause and repeat the process for each rep .

This method is highly effective, because your muscles are contracting as you're putting more tension on your muscle tissue. When you exert more pressure on those muscles, the outcome is that you will are able to increase the growth of your muscles.

Additionally it is recommended to begin each rep, you begin the exercise quickly and when you complete the rep, complete the exercise gradually.

It is also beneficial for cardio and muscle growth by doing a quick-paced, slow exercise many times that get your heart pumping and allows your muscles to expand .

Recently I was watching a huge man doing a 20kg chest press. I was struck by the uniqueness of this exercise was, since the man was constantly pausing after every rep. I was so intrigued by the workout that, after he had finished the exercise, I went up to him and told him, "I am deeply astonished that a pumped-up man like you can do an intense chest workout using an ungainly weight, so do you're one of the few guys who do not lift a lot of heavyweights in order to get large?".

He laughed and explainedthat "it does not matter what weight you are able to lift, it's all about the way you execute the exercise. When doing a chest exercise when you squeeze your chest for two seconds at the conclusion every rep while doing an intense amount of repetitions, your chest will expand".

I tried his method and I noticed that my muscles perform better. I felt pain due to the force and contraction I experienced from the chest exercises.

To sum it up If you employ the right method to your exercise routine, you can build muscle mass by using lightweight weights.

To swell your legs and quads doing squats with light weights, stop for two seconds while you lower and then go up slowly. Doing this can make your legs feel sore.

This is the same for deadlifts. In order to cause your lower back to explode when you lift your body up, stop and press your back for two seconds . Don't be fooled this technique is highly efficient.

The same goes when doing back exercises.

When you are bringing the weight closer the chest area, stop for two seconds. In essence, the most important thing is to complete the reps slow and in a controlled.

As stated that you can make use of one kettlebell for the chest flat and incline, as well as chest and chest decline exercises .

This can be accomplished by gripping the kettlebell's handle with both hands . From there, you're good to begin.

If you have a kettlebell, you may also push on both sides of your chest at the same time.

At first you could employ one hand on the kettlebell's handle to push to the chest's right hand. Once you do your reps after which, change to the left side to hold the handle in order to exercise on the lower left portion of the chest, and finish your repetitions.

You may even decide to alternate on between the chests on each side following each rep to increase intensity.

There are many ways to mix your workouts for your chest using just one kettlebell. It is up to you to determine the type of exercise that will work for you.

Personally, I like to change things up. I try all of these exercises to vary my workout and so to give my muscles a shock. This is because , when you do various exercises the body's body reacts to a different workout, which makes it more efficient.

Kettlebell Exercise

This photo illustrates me lifting a kettlebell that weighs 24kg for a chest exercise flat that targets the middle of the chest.

As you can see in the image, I performed this exercise in the ground . It is extremely effective because sitting on the ground strengthens and strengthens your skills. While lying on the floor the body is with your body straight and stationary . This allows you to concentrate more, and make the most results from this workout.

Chest Workout

When I go to training, I employ dumbbells for chest fly exercises. It is convenient since you can utilize both dumbbells to train both sides and the middle of your chest simultaneously.

The great thing is that you are able to only use one kettlebell to catch chest flies. This can be achieved by using both one of you to grasp the kettlebell's handle.

When your hand is gripping the handle, you can move it away from the chest area as far as you can. then, return the kettlebell back up to your chest . Repeat the steps with the same hand to finish the repetitions, or switch hands after each rep in order to effectively strengthen this part of your chest.

As you can see, I completed a chest incline that works the upper chest while on the floor.

Perhaps you're thinking about how to perform chest inclines in the ground since, for this kind of exercise it is recommended to use an adjustable bench that can slowly alter the position of the bench, so it is facing upwards.

You can do it in many ways. Instead of lying on your back completely the best thing could you do? to tilt your head slightly upwards so that the upper part that is your head directed towards the upwards.

It is vital to understand that this kind of exercise is challenging as the tilting of your body upwards can result in some stress on your body. The body isn't fully lying down, therefore it can be difficult to remain still. This can mean that when you are lifting your kettlebell it will not be moving in a straight line.

This exercise requires a high degree of skill, perseverance and consistent practice because one must be able to keep the body in a balanced state.

If you're not sure about your the body's natural balance, do not fret. By relying on self-belief, self-discipline, and commitment, this kind of exercise can be done.

But, if you don't like this kind of chest incline exercise There are other options.

If you're doing kettlebell exercises at home, get a chair allows you to move your body a little towards the upwards.

If you're able to find enough space in your home you could also make use of the wall to raise your body or make use of couch seating in your living space.

If you reside in a home with an outdoor garden, and you have steps, you could place your body on the steps where you lean your body up to perform an upward incline to your chest.

If, however, you do not like doing your workout at home or would like to change your preferred choice of training site from time-to-time you can use benches in parks.

In my Instagram posts , I utilized the bench at the park for my chest exercises.

Each of the methods I've listed will allow you to perform an incline-based chest press with a kettlebell that is placed on the floor.

Another chest exercise you can perform is a chest decline which works on the lower area of the chest.

What can I do to perform the lower chest exercise with kettlebells if I do not have an adjustable bench to lower?.

If there's will, there is a way.

It's an issue of thinking out of the box and coming up with an avenue.

I've mentioned before that you could utilize your couch or chair at home for an exercise for your chest. Similar is the case to a chest decline exercise.

Here's how:

Instead of tilting your body back instead, move your legs until they are close to the edge of the sofa or chair. Then, this allows your body to tilt down.

If your body is in this direction, you're now in a decline phase and are prepared to begin the chest drop.

Like the chest slope it is also possible to utilize your garden steps for the chest drop. It can be accomplished by putting both legs on the steps.

If you have space, you could have both feet in contact with the wall. It is important to make sure that they are touching the wall slightly higher since this allows your body to tilt downwards.

I also suggested that going to the park is an alternative for these types of exercises. If you're doing the chest drop it is possible to apply the same concept. If you can slide both your legs towards the top of the bench. you get great results from this exercise.

In my photo it is clear that I completed the chest exercise at the park, using the bench.

Shoulder Rakes

Utilize your hands to grasp those handles to the kettlebell in order to perform shoulder lifts, which work to the shoulders simultaneously.

As you can see in my photo I used a 24-kg Kettlebell to perform shoulder raises on the playground .

The usual method of doing shoulders raises at the gym would be to train with the dumbbells with each hand, working one shoulder at a time , then changing to the other hand to perform the other shoulder.

If you want to strengthen both shoulders simultaneously at the gym, you'd utilize two dumbbells and make sure they weigh the same.

It is still a good exercise since both shoulders are working simultaneously, that maximizes efficiency of time.

If I'm in the gym and doing an exercise for my shoulders, I employ both dumbbells of the same weight for your shoulder lifts.

The most appealing aspect of kettlebells is that you can use one kettlebell for on both shoulders simultaneously!

It is also possible to use two kettlebells with the same weight to strengthen both shoulders simultaneously So you have the option of doing that too.

To reap the maximum benefits of shoulder raises using just one kettlebell , it's essential to position yourself properly . Be sure that you have enough space when you move the kettlebell upwards and make sure that your body is in space to will have one leg in front and the other one behind.

133

Once you've properly positioned your body, you're now ready for this intense exercise.

Begin by holding the kettlebell's handle using both hands, making sure that you hold as tight the grip as you can. then place the kettlebells on your legs.

Breathe through and out, flex your power, and then use all of your strength and force to lift the kettlebell as high as you can.

Be sure to take a pause of 2 seconds, then lower your body slowly and climb up again in the fastest way you can using similar force.

Perform the most reps you can , and always aim at quality reps, not just quantity.

This kind of exercise will certainly hammer your shoulders since it is focused precisely on this region of the body. While you lift your shoulders to the highest level you can and more pressure is placed on the shoulders.

Furthermore, when you move fast and up and down this will have your heart rate running, making your workout an intense one that results in a great exercise routine.

This exercise will definitely build muscle and increase mass your shoulders.

Trapezius (Traps)

Utilize your hands to grasp those handles on the kettlebell in order to engage both of your traps simultaneously.

Like you see on my photo I was using my kettlebell of 24kg.

For this exercise to be effective, I grasped the kettlebell's handle using both hands and lowered the weight the highest I could to maximize the effectiveness the muscle.

When I was happy that I had lifted the kettlebell close to me as far as it was possible I followed the standard of pausing for 2 to 3 seconds, where I held the kettlebell high to my chest for a few seconds and then slowly lower it and then repeated the process until I was exhausted from the repetitions.

With Kettlebells I love the way I can increase my effectiveness as I work with both my traps at simultaneously.

It is also crucial to keep in mind that when you are at fitness, you may also utilize both hands to grasp the barbell and then perform the same exercise , working both traps at same at the same time.

But, only a single Kettlebell could accomplish this feat.

In my photo I'm also using the kettlebell to exercise the same muscle group however, the way I do it is slightly different. In this instance I'm shifting my shoulders, while using the kettlebells, and squeeze both shoulders.

Here, I aim to squeeze as long as I can , as this causes immense tension on my traps. This can blow your traps up and create that stunning shape that everyone hopes to have.

If you've got those lovely traps, it'll make your shoulders appear gorgeous. I've noticed that the traps are an important part of your muscles as they support the shape and appearance the shoulders. The traps are the backbone of your shoulders.

When I train in the gym, when doing shoulder shrugs, I'd need to utilize both dumbbells for this exercise. Then I'd need use the barbell. But with the help of a Kettlebell I'm getting impressive results.

More Shoulder Exercise

Utilize your hands to grip the kettlebell's face to perform shoulder presses either sitting or standing up, working both shoulders simultaneously .

The kind of exercise will be a surprise to many since a typical shoulder press requires at minimum 2 kettlebells or two dumbbells . Even 2 kettlebells , since I have observed popular shoulder presses using two kettlebells. In the normal course of my time at my gym I notice me performing shoulder presses, you'll be able to observe me using two dumbbells with the same weight. I was unable to exercise in the gym , and using just one kettlebell needed to be sacrificed. I had to think out of the box . In honest and

137

sincerity I was confident in the ability to do the shoulder press using just one kettlebell. I stood with my conviction that in this world, there's an almost always a way around any obstacle.

The moment when I realized that it was time to be honestwas when I began to figure out which kettlebell part is the one that carries the most weight . Okay, to help you to know what I'm talking about I began to hold different pieces of kettlebell in order to determine which kettlebell I felt had greater weight and had greater impact. I began to notice that the front of the kettlebell seemed heavier . From there I carefully grabbed the kettlebell, and then lifted it towards my chest. I'm not lying I felt the force when I carried it up to my chest, and I smiled that was a smile of triumph in discovering how to do the shoulder presses using just only one kettlebell, which could work both shoulders.

To begin I held my grip with a firm hold on the kettlebell and I gently pushed it up to the highest level I could for the first time to give me an idea of how the exercise would go . I stopped for a couple of minutes and then followed the method of gradually lifting the kettlebell until it was at my chest. I was pleased with the workout and became more comfortable with it, to the point that I kept doing the repetitions using this routine. I would highly recommend that you to try this exercise because it primarily concentrates on your shoulders, and places an intense amount of stress upon your shoulders. Take a look at my photo showing me using just the same kettlebell for an upper body press.

Chapter 12: 8 Week Training Plan

This is the beginning of the 8-week training program! Take advantage of the time spent training and concentrate on every movement Make your training as mindful as is possible.

If you're new to the sport to the sport, begin with lighter weights and gradually increase gradually over eight weeks. It is important to read reliable sources for demonstrations of movement and review your own movement to ensure you're performing your exercises in a safe way.

Each week will be comprised of endurance, strength, conditioning and endurance, and a few weeks also have the flow. I created four weekly complete workouts. It is possible to supplement your training with other activities such as rowing, running powerlifting, gymnastics, the jujitsu or kickboxing, or design your own workouts by using the extra workouts from Chapter 9.

Training Terminology

Through the course of training, you'll be exposed to the words below. Check this list as you require.

AMRAP AMRAP is "as as many sessions (and repetitions) as you can". In an AMRAP exercise, you'll do as hard as you can in the time you have to count down, and try to finish the most work you can within the time limit.

The EMOM acronym means "every minute of each minute". When you do an EMOM workout it is a good idea to start the next set of work at the beginning of each minute. You will then take all remaining time in the minute to take a break.

For Time An "for time" conditioning exercise is when you complete the exercise as fast as you can.

Rounds - A round in an exercise means that you repeat the same sequence of exercises for a set number of rounds. For instance the "5 round" workout is completed when all the movements of each round are completed five times.

Rep method This book follows a set reps and sets scheme. This means a four 6 workout is four sets of six repetitions. The workout appears like "10 10, 8 8 6 6, 6" will require that many reps, with rest between. Higher rep sets will have less weight than the lower rep sets.

Week 1

The first week is comprised of basic exercises and strength development. This will be the foundation of the eight-week program. Pay attention to the rep plan and start by using smaller weights, as you increase your weight over the course of the strength workout. This week's workout will include some of everything to help you become familiar with the various types of exercises we'll do.

Day 1

Strength:

Goblet Squat

10, 10, 10, 8, 8, 8, 6, 6, 6

Farmers carry

1 minute on and off for 10 minutes

Conditioning:

75 kettlebell swings

30 burpees

75 kettlebell swings

Day 2

Strength:

Single KB dl

5 8

Then:

Turkish get up:

5 3L/3R

Power Endurance:

Double kettlebell front racked walking lunges for 100 meters and back

*Reset and repeat

Day 3

Strength:

Double kettlebell press

10, 10, 8, 8, 4, 4, 2, 2

Conditioning:

1. Flow 1.

Two kettlebells on the floor

Hike to wash

Double front Squat

The front rack is a back-up for the thruster.

Reverse lunge each side

Bring kettlebells down to the floor.

Renegade row

Repeat 3 times

The exercise is completed in one round. stop for a moment and repeat 5 times.

Day 4

Strength:

Hike to wash

6 4l/4r

Conditioning:

4 rounds:

200m farmers carry

1 minute hang bar

20 air squats

Rest for 1 minute

Week 2

144

Day 1

Strength:

Double kettlebell Squat

5 10

15 push-ups per round.

Conditioning:

3 minutes:

5 goblet Squats

10 push-ups

1 minute of rest

3 minutes:

10 swings with kettlebells

30 double unders (50 single unders)

1 minute of rest

*Repeat entire sequence one time, for a total of sixteen minutes.

Day 2

Strength:

Single leg kettlebell Single leg kettlebell

5 10

EMOM at 10 mins

15 kettlebell swings

Conditioning:

4 rounds of time for each

10 goblet 10 squats

5 right side overhead press

10 goblets 10 goblets

5 left side overhead press

15 push ups

Day 3

Strength:

Double the KB press

5x6

Then:

Do 20 to 20 alternate Turkish workouts using moderate to low weight

Conditioning:

10 rounds

50 jump rope

10 push-up

10 goblets or mace Squat

Day 4

Strength:

Complex Snatch

Three times grab the right side from swing

3 right-hand swings

Transition to left

3 left side snatch snatch off the swing

3 swing

Then:

5 rounds:

10 alternating kettlebell figure 8

Conditioning:

50 swings of kb

200 jump rope

30 burpees

100 jump rope

15 pull-ups

50 jump rope

Week 3

Week 3 begins with Turkish wear-ups and windmills. They are difficult and multi-skilled exercises therefore, start slowly and use less weight when this is the first time you've completed these movements. We'll finish this week with an old-fashioned Tabata routine exercise. Do your best and push hard!

Day 1

Strength:

Turkish get-up

4 3r/3l

*use the same weight as the previous week

Then:

Kettlebell windmill

3 5l/5r

Power endurance:

Continue to carry 50m during 20 minutes. Recover as you need to.

Day 2

Strength:

Double KB Squat

5 8

Then:

6 rounds:

8l/8r kettlebell row

15 push-ups

Take a break as you need between sets

Then:

6 rounds:

10 weighted step-ups

10 swings with kettlebells

Day 3

Strength:

Seesaw press

6 8

Then:

Floor press

5 5 x

Conditioning:

2. Flow

1l kettlebell hike, clean and tidy

3L swing cleaning

3l overhead press

1r kettlebell hike, clean

3rd swing cleaning

3r overhead press

Rest : 30 seconds, repeat 10 times

Day 4

Strength:

Single kettlebell to grab

Gradually increase the weight over several sets:

8 5l/5r

Then:

Five sets of ME weighted pull-ups

*ME = Maximum Effort Max effort means that you perform as many repetitions as you can in a set until you are able to not continue.

Conditioning:

The following is a list of the 20-minute on/ off times.

Squat

Squat

Swing

Swing

Clean and press

Clean and press

Deadlift

Week 4

This week will include lots of kettlebell exercise. Make use of this time to train your mind and build functional strength and stability.

The squat workout will require you do 3 single sided front squats before moving the kettlebell back for three back squats, then switch sides.

Day 1

Strength:

Single arm deadlift

6 4l/4r

*Use a large weight and concentrate on stability

Power endurance:

2 mile run

400m sandbag carry

30 burpees

30 pull-ups

200m kettlebells are used by farmers to carry

30 Squats

30 push-ups

2 mile run

Day 2

Strength:

Single kb Squat Complex

Complete eight sets:

3rd front squat

3rd back squat

3l front 3l front

3l back 3l back

Then:

5 x 5 sandbags clean and press

Conditioning:

Flow 3.

Start in hike position

Double Kb swing

Double kb clean , press and clean

KB drop to the floor

Sprawl kettlebell off

Double KB deadlift

2 Push-ups off the the KB handle

Renegade row left/right

Return to your hike position

Perform two times then rest, repeating entire process 6 times

Day 3

Strength:

Single arm overhead press

6 4l/4r

Conditioning:

12 minutes EMOM

15 KB swings

15 sit ups

15 ring dips

If you don't have access to rings, you can perform normal dips. If do not have the capacity to perform bar dips you can substitute 20 push-ups

Power endurance:

10 minutes AMRAP

50m drag of sled

Day 4

Strength:

Single clean

As many quality reps as you can within the 10 minutes you have to complete the exercise

Three left hands, then swing the other hand to switch hands 3 right.

Conditioning:

8 rounds

10 kb deadlifts

15 pull-ups

20 push-ups

Week 5

Day 1

Strength:

Double overhead kettlebell squat

10, 10, 8, 8, 5, 5, 5

*Do 10 push-ups as well as 10 chin-ups in between sets.

Conditioning:

4 rounds:

200-meter farmers carry

10 sandbag clean

10 burpees

1 minute hang bar

Day 2

Strength:

6 rounds:

6 double swings

4 double snatch

Then:

Weighted lunges

5 12

Conditioning:

8 minutes EOM:

15 Kettlebell swing

Day 3

Strength:

Clean and press

5, 5, 5, 3, 3, 3, 1, 1

Then:

Floor press

5 10

Then:

Weighted step-ups

6 20

Day 4

Strength:

Kettlebell windmill

6 3L/3R

Conditioning:

1 minute for each exercise:

Kettlebell Two hand row

Double kettlebell clean until squatting

Sandbag shouldering

Pull-ups

Abmat sit-ups

*Repeat the exercise for one minute. Repeat to complete five sets

Week 6

We've got another brand new move this week the single press with farmers hold. To perform this exercise, you must place an kettlebell while in the farmer's carry position while pressing the second kettlebell overhead from an upright position on the front rack. We also offer strength endurance exercises using AMRAP Sled Drags.

Day 1

Strength:

6 rounds:

10 goblets 10 goblets

*10 push-ups and 5 chin ups between each round of strength

Conditioning:

3 rounds:

Run 400 meters

21 kettlebell swings

12 pull-ups

Day 2

Strength:

Double KB deadlift

8, 8, 8, 6, 6, 6

Then:

Romanian deadlift

4x8

Conditioning:

Flow 3.

Start in hike position

Double Kb swing

Double kb clean , press and clean

KB drop to the floor

Sprawl kettlebell off

Double KB deadlift

2 Push-ups off the the handle of the KB

Renegade row left/right

Return to your hike position

Do this 2 times, and then finish the entire flow sequence six times in total.

Day 3

Strength:

Single arm press Farmers

6x6

Conditioning:

5 rounds, work 30 seconds, rest 30 seconds:

Kettlebell is able to swing

Ball hits the floor

Sit ups

Walking lunges (weighted if you desire)

Day 4

Strength:

Weighted step-ups

5 10/10/10

Then:

Pull ups with weighted handles

5 ME

*ME = Max Effort max effort is the ability to do as many repetitions as you can in a set until you are able to stop.

Power endurance:

20-minute AMRAP

Dragsled

10 burpees to start of each 2 minute

Week 7

Day 1

Strength:

10 rounds:

159

5 double KB squats, 5 double KB thrusters to 5 thruster

*90 second break between sets

Flow:

Flow 1.

Two kettlebells on the floor

Hike to wash

Double front Squat

The front rack is a back-up for the thruster.

Reverse lunge each side

Bring kettlebells down to the floor.

Renegade row

Repeat 3 times

This is the end of 1 round. stop for a moment and repeat 5 times.

Day 2

Strength:

6 rounds:

With 2 kettlebells

1 Hike clean up to 2 swings clean

5 thruster

Conditioning:

4 rounds:

15 goblet 15 goblets

200m farmer transports

Day 3

Strength:

10 rounds:

2L 2, 2R Kettlebell push press and clean

4 Pull-up

:20 sec. Rest

Then:

See-saw press

5x5l/5r

Conditioning:

45 seconds of working time/minute rest

Kettlebell swing

Push-up

Day 4

Strength:

8 rounds:

10 Floor press

5 dips

5 chin-up

Conditioning:

21-15-9-15-21:

Ball smash

Squat and jump

Sit-up

*30 jump ropes between rounds

Week 8

Our last week! Maintain the intensity.

Day 1

Strength:

Goblet Squat

5 8

Then:

Front rack double kettlebell walking lunge

4 20

Conditioning:

Then, alternate EMOM every 10 mins

Even minutes:

20 swings

Odd minutes:

15 burpees

Day 2

Strength:

Single leg dl

8 6l/6r

Conditioning:

AMRAP 10 minutes

10 deadlifts

400m run

Day 3

Strength:

8 rounds:

3r snatch

3r press

3l Snatch

3l press

Then:

Weighted step-ups

5 20

Conditioning:

2 times:

AMRAP 3 minutes:

5 goblets 5 goblets

10 push-ups

Rest for 1:00 Then

AMRAP 3 minutes:

10 swings with kettlebells

60 jump rope

Rest 11:30

Day 4

Strength:

8 rounds:

4l/4r row

4l/4r floor press

Then:

8 minutes EMOM:

15 swings with kettlebells

Conditioning:

2. Flow

One kettlebell on the floor

Hike to swing

Swing to cleanse

Clean and hygienic to the overhead press

Press your head to squat, then press the overhead to thruster

Hand change to the person who is swung

Repeat on opposite side.

Rest and repeat for a total of reps of 10 minutes

Checking for

What do you think?

I hope that after the eight weeks of exercise you're feeling stronger and ready to face new challenges with confidence and endurance. If you've completed the conditioning part it's likely that you'll feel an increase in your aerobic fitness.

Utilize exercises such as the goblet squat, or a single kettlebell deadlifts to measure and then retest your strength levels as you progress. Find out how far you can achieve and keep track of your how far you've come over time. Go back to the workouts from this guide and observe how much quicker and easier you are able to complete these exercises.

Chapter 13: Beginners, Intermediate, and Advanced Level Kettlebell Workout plan

As we said earlier, it's important to only engage in kettlebell workouts that your body is able to handle. For beginners, this means you shouldn't do intense kettlebell workouts. To avoid injury, there are three levels.

Starter Kettlebell Workouts

This exercise has two main goals: to increase your strength and endurance in large muscles. It also helps to improve your cardiovascular performance. The recommended duration is between 15 minutes and 45 minutes. You should also perform three circuits in a single workout. This is shown in this table.

Kettlebell

Exercises Length

Important Notes

Kettlebell Swing 1-1-3

Minutes

Move the kettlebell.

Half off the Kettlebell Glasset

Up to 3

Minutes

Kettlebell One-arm Row 3-3

Minutes

Make sure you have your chest exposed. Keep your elbows down.

1-arm Overhead Press

Minutes This is an alternative to our common bench press.

These are the most common. However, the overhead presse requires a complex wrist and arm movement.

Kettlebell Halo 1-3

Minutes

Keep your lower back in place and keep it at the pivot

Intermediate Level Kettlebell Training

This level is intended to build muscular strength and endurance. Its three times more demanding than the beginner level and will work the muscles threex as hard. It is important for improving cardiovascular performance. This session takes 40 minutes. At this level, there are three circuits.

Kettlebell exercise length/number

repetitions Important Notes

Kettlebell Swing 12-15 minute Here, your hips and glutes must drive the kettlebell forward. Instead of using your arms, you need to use your hips. The trick is to keep your hips and glutes engaged throughout the entire exercise.

exercise

KettlebellOnearm Row 8-10

Repeats per side

exercise

One-armKettlebell FloorPress 8-10

Multiple repetitions per side

Keep your feet together with the kettlebell, pressing in the upward direction.

Kettlebell Turkish Take Up 6-8 repetitions on each side. This is a complex exercise that involves several movements. The most important movement in this exercise is to move your leg forward so it can support you.

That you require while in a lunge pose

Kettlebell Goblet Squat 12-15 minute Go as low to your heart rate as you can, but don't let your tailbone get in the way of your butt.

Advanced Level Kettlebell Training

The advanced kettlebell level is appropriate for those who have completed both the first and second levels. They have sufficient flexibility and muscular strength to perform the advanced workouts.

This level will not only increase muscle endurance and muscular strength but it will also pay closer attention to strengthening your core and increasing your cardio capacity. This level should be done for at least 40 minutes each session. Three circuits are recommended per workout.

Kettlebell exercise length/number

repetitions Important Notes

Kettlebell Windmill 8-10 repetitions Per Side. Since this is a very challenging exercise, you should start with lightweight kettlebells. To ensure that the kettlebell is raised overhead, you must keep your focus on the weight.

You ensured proper shoulder alignment

The Kettlebell Deadlift - Try to do at least 15 reps. Here, engage your core and tighten your glutes. Keep your arms straight while raising the body. Also, push your feet up. This is the best way. Do not pull the kettlebells up with your arms. Instead, let the kettlebells move naturally along with your body.

to a standing position

Kettlebell Split Jerk: Start with 4-5 reps per leg and then increase the number to 8-10 according to your fitness level.

Increases

Kettlebell Pistol Stain 4-5 per leg first, then build it up to 8-10 in your fitnesslevel

Increases

Keep your kettlebell clean 15-18 times Keep your knees bent when you are reaching down to grip the handle. Also, make sure to keep your thumb back. In rack position, the kettlebell should rest on one side of your body. The other side should rest on your forearm.

The chest level is where it should be.

Chapter 14: Personalize It!

This is a great place for beginners to get started with kettlebell training.

MAKE IT YOUR OWN

Mixing and matching single exercises can be a great way of keeping your body active and avoiding boredom. It's easy to customize your workout by choosing the exercises you love and the areas you want.

CHOOSE A FOCUS

To create your own personalized kettlebell program, you must first determine the goals and focus of the workout. There are four possible areas to focus:

Upper body

Lower body

Core

Full-body

A variety of workouts can be created based upon different areas of focus, for different days of each week.

EXERCISE SELECTION

Your area of focus and your goals will guide the exercises you choose. You can use many kettlebell moves to target different muscles in your body. The majority of exercises will have a single focus. Take advantage of the handy list of exercises in each chapter to choose exercises based on the main focus of your workout plan.

A full-body plan doesn't necessarily have to be limited to exercises like the kettlebell swivel, which is often referred to as a 'full-body' workout. It's possible to mix up different moves to get a more comprehensive workout.

CARDIO VS. STRENGTH

It is important to choose whether you want your focus to be cardio or strength-based when setting a workout goal.

A strength-based plan will allow you to lift slower and with a heavier weight. If you want to build strength, you should pick a weight you can only lift for 10 repetitions. This will make it more difficult for your

174

muscles and will result in a shorter workout.

Cardio-focused moves will be those that give you good cardio while not increasing your weight. Your heart rate will rise faster and you can train for longer hours without fatigue.

REPETITIONS and INTERVALS

You can categorize each workout as either a repetition or an interval-based. A repetition-based work out would require that each exercise be repeated and set for a certain number of times. Interval-based training will have each exercise performed for a specified amount of times before moving on to the next.

Of course, repetition-based plans work well for strength training. Interruption-based plans work better for cardio. There is still plenty of room to experiment when creating your workouts.

EXERCISE REQUEST

As important as the kettlebell exercises themselves, is how they are placed within your training plan. Combining similar exercises that work the same part of your body can lead to muscle fatigue. In order to allow your muscles to rest, alternate exercises that target the upper, core, or lower body.

THE REPETITION PLAN

To create a repetition-based program for your workout, you must first decide what outcome you want.

Muscle endurance

Muscle size

Muscle power and strength

The goal determines the number and length of repetitions, sets, rest times, and set duration.

Muscle endurance

Increase your muscle mass to do more reps faster and for longer periods of time without tiring.

Light weight

High reps, 12-20+

Sets: 3 - 5

Retired: 30- 60 seconds to 2 minutes, with a break of 1 – 2 minutes between sets

Size of your Muscles

Build bigger muscles.

Heavy weight

Medium reps: 6 - 12

Sets: 3 - 5

More rest 60 to 90 seconds. You can also take up 2 to 3 minutes between sets.

Stärke and Power

Strengthen your muscles without making them bigger

Very heavy weight

Low reps 1 - 5.

Sets: 3 - 5

Long rest: between sets, up to 3 minutes to 5 minutes

THE INTERVAL PLAN

You'll need to distinguish between active phases (or resting phases) when you make an interval training plan. Active phases represent the time that is spent on the exercise. Resting phases are the time between active and rest phases.

As a rule, active phases should be between 30 seconds and 2 minutes. Resting phases should be between 10 seconds and 30 secs. Your level and conditioning will determine how long each phase lasts. Before you begin to create an interval plan, make sure you test how long you can comfortably do the exercise. Also, find out how much time it takes to recover from the active phase. You can adjust your interval workout based on this information.

HOW MANY EXERCISES

It can be difficult to decide which kettlebell exercise to include in your routine. But there is a guideline for how many you should include. A kettlebell works out many muscles in one exercise. This means that your workouts should contain fewer exercises than those where you are focusing on smaller or single muscle groups. In order to achieve a full-body, effective workout, you should pick three to five exercises for the upper and lower body.

CHOOSING AN WEIGHT

It all depends on your goals as well as your abilities. It is also an exercise in trial and error. It is best to start light and not go overboard. It's better for you to see that you could have performed more reps and used a lighter weight than to finish a work out and call an ambulance.

You can start by starting with a lighter-weight weight, and then work your way up to the recommended number of reps. Once the workout is over, evaluate how you feel. You can increase your weight or increase the reps/sets until you find the right balance.

In interval-based training, you should be lighter and have shorter active phase and longer rest phases. After your first workout, you will be able to assess whether or not you need an increase in weight, active phases, and decreased rest phases.

Only by learning to experiment with the variables and listening carefully to your body, you will be able to identify the issues and create a customized workout plan for you.

HOW DO YOU INCREASE WEIGHT, REPS/SETS?

There is no definitive way to increase the kettlebell weight or the number or repetitions of sets you perform. This is a personal decision that you have to make.

REPS & SETS

Kettlebell weight increase can lead to big leaps in weight. This can make it difficult to decide whether to lift the kettlebell weight. It is usually easier to increase the number repetitions or sets before increasing the weight. Here's how.

You can move your workouts using the beginner, intermediate and advanced workouts described earlier in chapters.

Start with the recommended body weight as detailed in Chapter 3. Start with the smallest number possible of reps. In this example, it would be eight repetitions for three sets. To get more comfortable, you can increase your reps by 1 for each set to 9 reps for three-sets. Continue increasing your reps to reach the maximum number for a set. Continue increasing the number and size of your sets.

If you find it difficult or impossible to increase the sets to the maximum recommendation reps, reduce the reps back eight and increase them instead. Once you have reached your maximum set, you can begin to increase the number of reps per each set.

When you can perform five sets with 10 reps each comfortably, it is time to think about increasing your weight.

WEIGHT

Kettlebell weight increases are much more significant than the smaller incremental gains available with traditional weightlifting such as dumbbells. Barbells and dumbbell weight plates come in sizes of 500 g/1lb. However, kettlebells offer a

4-kg/9-lb weight increase. However, it is not a decision that should be taken lightly.

Perfecting your form is key to gaining weight. Once you have perfected this form, your decision on how to build muscle will be influenced.

If you're looking to improve muscle endurance, consider increasing your body weight. A seamless set of 20+ reps is the best way to go. You shouldn't feel exhausted at the conclusion of a set.

If you're looking to bulk up your muscles or increase your size, consider increasing your kettlebell weight. When you can do 6-12 repetitions per sets, this will give you the maximum number without feeling fatigued or compromise form.

Consider increasing your kettlebell strength to increase power and endurance. A kettlebell should weigh 3 to 5 repetitions for each exercise. This will give you the best chance of completing as many sets as you want without getting tired.

If you have any questions regarding how to increase your body weight, it is a good idea for a trainer to help you. Because of the increased weight when you go from one kettlebell option to the next, there is always the possibility of injury. To speak with a trainer you don't have to visit a gym. There are numerous forums where personal trainers offer their expertise to those who are just starting out in fitness. Many trainers or instructors also have websites that allow you to reach them. Always remember to contact your instructor or trainer if in doubt.

Conclusion

A kettlebell makes a great tool for any workout. This is due to its unique shape which allows for multiple exercises. These are all good for the body. It is important to order the exercises in a way that allows the individual to get the maximum benefit from the time they spend. Beginers should include Turkish getups swings, lunges or Turkish get-ups in their weekly workouts. First, it is important to maintain balance with kettlebells. Then you can switch to high-intensity exercise. This is why the swing is the most important exercise. It should not be mixed in with other exercises. If an individual attempts to push too hard or progress too quickly, there's a risk of injury. This could result in the end of all exercise. It is recommended that you keep your workouts simple and take the time to master each exercise. This will allow the body to grow and change as it progress.

www.ingramcontent.com/pod-product-compliance
Lightning Source LLC
Chambersburg PA
CBHW060329030426
42336CB00011B/1270